P9-DFF-014

How to use natural cures

to reverse respiratory ailments

The

Respiratory

Solution

REVISED EDITION

Finally, relief from

asthma, bronchitis, mold,

sinus attacks, allergies,

sore throats, colds, and flu

Dr. Cass Ingram

Knowledge House
Buffalo Grove, Illinois

Copyright March 2003, Knowledge House

First revised edition
All rights reserved. No part of this publication may be
reproduced without prior written consent from the publisher.
Printed in Canada

Disclaimer: This book is not intended as a substitute for medical
diagnosis or treatment. Anyone with a serious disease should con-
sult a physician before initiating any change in treatment or before
beginning any new treatment.

For ordering information call (800) 243-5242 or for overseas
orders call (847) 473-4700. To send a fax: (847) 473-4780. To
send an e-mail: droregano@aol.com. For more information about
the products mentioned in this book see the Web site, Oreganol.com.

ISBN: 1-931078-07-6

Table of Contents

Introduction

Respiratory diseases are among the most pervasive of all medical conditions. It seems that virtually everyone suffers from some type of respiratory complaint. Sinus problems, colds, flu, sore throat, scratchy throat, hoarseness, irritable nose, runny nose, itchy eyes, allergies, shortness of breath, asthma, hay fever, earaches: everyone occasionally suffers from one or more of these conditions.

Today, respiratory problems are an international epidemic. Continuously, significant outbreaks occur throughout the world. The fact is during the appropriate seasons the risks for such outbreaks are constant. What's more, the incidence of asthma, bronchitis, persistent cough, pneumonia, sinusitis, and emphysema is increasing astronomically. Diseases previously regarded as controlled or eradicated have reappeared. Even whooping cough has made a comeback.

Respiratory illnesses are a vast dilemma: billions are affected not just yearly but also daily. However, there is no need to suffer endlessly from such conditions. There is a cure, and the cure is from nature. In contrast, drugs fail to cure respiratory illnesses. Asthma and emphysema are excellent examples. No drug has been found to cure them. In fact, the drugs typically used for the conditions aggravate them. In contrast, natural medicines are capable of curing respiratory illnesses, because they greatly aid the function of the lungs. What's more, there are a number of natural substances which, if taken regularly, may prevent the occurrence of lung or respiratory diseases.

In order to comprehend why respiratory infections are so common the function of the lungs must be reviewed. The purpose of the lungs is to process air. They are an elastic organ capable of drawing in air. Once the air enters it is filtered. Here, the lungs sort the good from the bad, the healthy from the toxic, and the clean from the filthy. They are a type of living filter system with the ability to expunge anything undesirable. This means they are able to cleanse the air to a large degree before it enters the blood. If that cleansing function fails, disease develops. The lungs also sort the air, absorbing only the life-giving gas known as oxygen, while expelling all others. The air is filtered not by the lungs but by the remainder of the respiratory tree, including the tonsils, sinuses, nostrils, and bronchial tubes.

When they are overwhelmed as a result of the inhalation of toxins, germs, or other debris, the result is inflammation. The toxins in fact activate the lungs' immune system, leading to swelling and inflammation. This may result in difficulty breathing, mucous build-up, and/or cough. The swelling and inflammation, if unresolved, breeds further infection, because congestion of the tissues aids in microbial growth. To resolve this condition the toxins and/or germs must be purged from the lungs. Throughout this book the proper approach to achieve this will be described.

The lungs are the largest organs in the respiratory system, and they are the primary ones involved in respiratory diseases. Other respiratory organs include the throat (trachea), bronchial passages, sinuses, nasal passages, mouth, and ear canals.

Today, there is a greater vulnerability for the development of diseases of the lungs and other respiratory organs than ever before in history. The air that is breathed is never clean. It is so heavily polluted that lung damage is inevitable. In the Western world in particular no one can escape. There is extensive air pollution in every city and, in fact, every corner of the globe. Even the air in the high mountains is polluted. Obviously, some regions are more polluted than others, the worst being major metropolitan areas such as Los Angeles, New York City, Chicago, Rome, Istanbul, Cairo, Tokyo, London, Ankara, or Athens. Yet, no region is pollution-free. The fact is the toxic effects of noxious air are inescapable.

Global warming aggravates the dilemma. A hot atmosphere accelerates the toxicity of airborne pollutants. Plus, dry weather increases the levels of toxic particles, since rain is needed to flush them from the air. Rain may remove the vast majority of air pollutants. Thus, in drought-like conditions air quality worsens significantly.

Deforestation also increases the risks for respiratory pollution. Trees are the primary means for the removal of noxious carbonic gases, like carbon dioxide and carbon monoxide, from the atmosphere. Thus, trees are nature's air filters. They aggressively detoxify carbon dioxide and similar gases. Carbonic gases are categorically respiratory poisons. What's more, the destruction of the rain forest has accelerated the release of certain germs into the atmosphere. For instance, currently, across the globe mold counts are at the highest level ever recorded.

The question is how can the lungs and other organs be protected from this toxicity? Certainly, drugs merely increase tissue toxicity, so they are of no value in lung protection. Thus, it is necessary to resort to natural medicines for the solution. Yet, the question is which foods, supplements, vitamins, minerals, spices, and herbs offer the most significant protection? Plus, which herbs or plant extracts are potent enough to halt respiratory symptoms and/or reverse disease?

The cells within the human body are made of natural substances. The mechanisms in which they operate are in concert with nature. The internal components of the cells, that is their living machinery, thrive on natural compounds. In contrast, such machinery is disrupted and even destroyed by synthetic, that is man-made, compounds. Synthetic substances readily destroy cells. Natural substances build them.

The lungs are highly delicate. Synthetic, toxic chemicals readily harm them. Natural chemicals, such as the substances found in food, herbs, and spices, boost lung function. Thus, the use of the natural pharmacy is the only reasonable solution for preventing and/or curing respiratory diseases.

The respiratory system is a combination of organs, which function as a unit. It includes the lungs, bronchial tubes, throat, sinuses, mouth, and even the ear canals. Of course, the lungs are the largest and most significant component. The lungs contain billions of tiny cells, known as alveoli. They have a vast surface area and, thus, act as a potential breeding ground for germs.

Complaints of the respiratory system are the primary reason for doctor visits. There are hundreds of respiratory conditions, some minor and some serious. A partial list of these conditions includes colds, flu, croup (in children), asthma, bronchitis, pneumonia, pleurisy, congestive heart failure, sinusitis, post nasal drip, sinus headache, runny nose, laryngitis, hoarseness, sore throat, tonsillitis, emphysema, and earaches.

Usually, respiratory conditions cause transitory symptoms. People are accustomed to the fact that sudden symptoms, such as cough, sore throat, congestion, runny nose, sinus pressure, sneezing fits, fever, chills, etc., rapidly disappear. However, if the condition is untreated and/or neglected, a chronic illness may develop. Some respiratory illnesses are lethal: for instance, asthma and pneumonia. In hospitalized patients pneumonia is a major cause of death, particularly for cancer patients and those with suppressed immunity. In fact, thousands of cancer patients die yearly from this seemingly preventable disease. Emphysema is often fatal, as are certain rather remote lung diseases such as asbestosis, berylliosis, and silicosis.

Cancer is perhaps the most feared of all respiratory illnesses. It is a devastating disease, and, once it is diagnosed, it usually results in a rather rapid death. It may attack any part of the respiratory system, although it most commonly develops in the lungs. However, throat cancer is an epidemic in Westernized countries, largely as a consequence of tobacco smoking. Here is another example of how man-made toxics are destroying people. In smokers lung cancer is the primary cause of death, and in medicine there is no known cure. However, the consequences can be positive, that is if the individual utilizes natural medicine in concert with medical care. Even with cancer the lungs can heal, that is if they are provided with the proper nutrients and are treated with the appropriate herbal tonics. The point is never give up hope. Natural medicines can come to the rescue.

There is yet another reason the lungs increase the vulnerability: they are the primary portal of entry for a wide range of poisons. They are the most readily accessible of all pathways by which dangerous substances can enter the body. This is because whatever is deeply inhaled into the lungs may also readily be absorbed into the general circulation, that is into the blood and lymph. A good example is anthrax. This is a germ which normally causes illnesses, but not fatalities. The fatalities are caused mainly by the biological form, the one made by the military-industrial complex. This war-grade anthrax was made specifically to kill and to do so quickly and in vast numbers. If the entire quota of anthrax stored in the U. S. stockpiles was released throughout the continental United

States, if unprotected, virtually every North American would die. Anthrax kills through inhalation, that is through the lungs. The fact is the direct inhalation of anthrax spores, especially the weaponized variety, usually results in death.

The likelihood of mass destruction from a rare germ like anthrax is minimal. The more significant causes of epidemics and, therefore, potentially thousands of deaths are more universal germs, like the flu virus, strep, or TB. Anthrax, Hantavirus, West Nile virus, and similar rare germs will always cause their share of deaths. However, the more serious epidemics will be caused by germs that are more widespread such as influenza, staph, strep, Candida albicans, mycoplasma, mycobacteria, flu virus, and molds. These are everyday germs found everywhere. Such germs cause both acute and chronic infections, and many cause significant chronic disease. What's more, they are nearly always found on or in people, continuously. These are the germs of global epidemics that will likely cause the majority of deaths and disabilities in the future. The fact is a global pandemic is inevitable.

This is not to underestimate the powers of the more bizarre germs. Untold numbers of lung and respiratory infections are caused by such germs, and, thus, their role must always be considered in diagnosing or treating the condition. In fact, all types of germs must be considered in order to properly address the true cause of each illness. For more information about which germs may be involved in a given condition see Chapter 4.

Even so, there is a need to simplify the treatment of respiratory diseases. What is needed are agents which neutralize the major factors which cause such diseases. Thus, there is a need for a universal antidote, in fact, a universal germicide. Such an agent must reverse the toxicity of germs, allergens, and pollutants. Incredibly, these are the very agents with which an entire category of living creatures must contend every day, that is the plant kingdom. The trees, shrubs, grasses, herbs, and food plants have continuously adapted mechanisms to survive insults by the aforementioned agents. Their mechanism is to produce chemicals, which act to neutralize any toxicity.

Have you ever wondered how plants, such as the trees which line a busy interstate highway, survive despite being constantly exposed to pollutants? They do so by producing special substances known as *phytochemicals*. The purpose of these substances is to help the plants combat stress, including the stress from pollutants as well as germs. Today, it is possible to extract such chemicals and use them for personal protection. In the plant kingdom there is a medicine for virtually any illness (a statement originally attributed to the Prophet Muhammad). This is a highly positive approach, completely opposite to the typical medical attitude, which is there is no cure. The prophetic approach indicates that if an individual is ill, he/she should never lose hope. Somewhere in nature there is a cure. It is a question of discovering it. Thus, the challenge is finding the appropriate "medicine" and determining how it should be used. It is the challenge of finding the individual who can provide the proper guidance and or means of administering such a cure. The information in this book helps solve this issue, that is it provides the appropriate plant medicines required to reverse respiratory complaints and to protect the lungs and other organs from toxic and/or microbial insults.

Chapter 1

The Breathing Mechanism

Breathing is an automatic process. No one has to think about it. The only time it stops is with death. The oxygen in the air is nourishment for the body. Oxygen is equally as important, in fact, more important, than food or water. People have survived up to a month without food and a week or more without water. However, without air it is possible only to survive a few minutes. Thus, the inhalation of air is the most critical of all body processes.

Through an automatic process controlled by the brain air is inhaled into the lungs. Quickly, it reaches the tiny cells, that is the alveoli, located throughout the lung tissue. The alveoli act to deliver the oxygen from the air into the blood. This oxygen is then captured by the red blood cells, which transport it through the blood and ultimately deliver it to the cells. The inhalation of air can be inhibited, that is by stress or poor posture. However, it is impossible to stop, except by death.

The lungs are a magnificent set of organs, which defy even science's understanding. How is it that such a system can turn air into the key source of cellular nutrition? How does this system operate continuously, performing its functions untold millions of times without seemingly wearing out? This is an utter marvel of nature, one that could only be attributed to a higher power.

Any basic review of their anatomy and function makes it evident that the lungs are perfectly designed. Therefore, it is reasonable to presume that they were designed by a Power that is unfathomable. Many people, even top scientists, might consider that over time such a refined system could evolve, apparently on its own. Yet, when carefully reviewing its grand structure it is seemingly impossible to believe that such a refined, complex organ system could develop simply through chance or mere evolution. The fact is the lungs are perfectly configured for processing air and converting it into a usable form. Truly, this is a marvel. Yet, despite the refinement of their function it is rare to find these organs operating in an optimal condition. Due to a variety of factors, such as pollution, poor posture, cigarette smoking, poor nutrition, etc., the function of the lungs can be greatly compromised. Thus, serious malfunction and even disease may develop. Yet, the lungs greatly resist such toxicity. However, ultimately, if the toxic insults are continuous, the resistance of the lungs is weakened, and, thus, a wide range of disorders may result. Thus, it is crucial to keep these organs in the most optimal condition possible.

An old Reader's Digest book, *Our Human Body: Its Wonders and Care,* provides an excellent overview of the lungs. J. D. Radcliff notes that human beings subject the lungs to a wide range of insults. For instance, he describes how slumping, sitting in a sloppy manner in soft chairs, cramping the body while sitting, etc., all impair their ability to keep us healthy. Smog, gasoline fumes, car exhaust, cigarette smoke, and industrial chemicals, as well as fumes from household cleaners and pesticides, damage these delicate organs on contact. Incredibly, the lungs are inflated half a billion times in a lifetime, which amounts to a massive amount of strain on such a fine organ system. Obviously, the lungs are more durable than any man-made machine, which could never withstand so many repetitions. Yet, this natural function, that is the natural "wear and tear" from mere breathing, is far from the major issue. It is the toxic insults that reach the lungs that cause the greatest degree of damage.

The lungs are a highly delicate system and, thus, are exceptionally vulnerable to toxicity. They would go into shock if they were directly and immediately exposed to pollutants or particulate matter as well as to extremes in air temperature. This dilemma is solved by the nose, which conditions the air and filters particulate matter. Every breath may deliver a potentially lethal amount of dust particles as well as allergens and microbes. Here again, the nasal passages, as well as sinuses, act as a buffer, filtering noxious items and producing mucous to lubricate, cleanse, trap, and condition. The mucous is a type of sticky compound, which traps any dust that passes over it, much like a warm gluey surface. Obviously, if dust is constantly being trapped, with time this accumulates and could clog the system. However, in one of its immense miracles the body has its own "street cleaners": the cilia, tiny hair-like projections with their own independent sweeping power, helping to cleanse the tissue linings and mucous of dust and other particulate matter.

The lungs have a vast blood supply. This is so that the red blood cells can mix readily with the air. The red cells contain a complex molecule called hemoglobin. It is the hemoglobin which traps oxygen so it can be transported to the cells and organs.

Everyone knows that blood is red. However, in certain areas the blood appears dark blue or purple. This is the blood inside veins. It is the same blood. However, this purplish blood is depleted of oxygen. Plus, it is high in carbon dioxide. When the venous blood is returned to the lungs, the oxygen is replenished and carbon dioxide is expelled. In other words, oxygen makes blood red. That is why the blood of people on oxygen tanks is unusually bright red.

Oxygen is crucial for sustaining health. It is the most vital life force. Without it all life must cease. In contrast, carbon dioxide is a cellular poison. If it accumulates in excess, life ceases. It is crucial that the body receives plenty of oxygen, while expelling as much carbon dioxide as possible. The purpose of breathing is to draw in sufficient oxygen and drive out the carbon dioxide. Anything which impairs breathing, such as spinal disease, abdominal illnesses, poor posture, stress, lung disease, medications, etc., diminishes health by impairing oxygen intake and increasing carbon dioxide retention.

The lungs are crucial for cleansing the tissues. Exhaled gases contain a wide range of toxins, that is the various waste products, from cellular metabolism. *Physiology and Hygiene*, published in 1900, describes the dangers of this toxicity. The authors note that the waste gases from human exhalation are not only poisonous to the individual, but also to the group. Have you ever noticed a heavy or foul "human smell" in closed rooms with large numbers of humans? That smell isn't body odor; it is the odor of foul human gases from exhaled air.

It is crucial to have a healthy breathing mechanism to maintain superior health. If the breathing process is disrupted, overall health will suffer. In order to do so take deep breaths often and exhale thoroughly. Healthy breathing is an art which must be practiced. Incredibly, we often forget to breathe and rarely take the time to take a deep breath. The fact is relaxed deep breathing is such a powerful technique that it may by itself result in an immediate improvement in health.

With every breath there is a trade: oxygen for carbon dioxide and other waste gases. This is what sustains life. If this trade is imbalanced, ill health results. If it is severely disrupted, death may result.

Yet, to breathe pure oxygen is dangerous, except for very short periods of time. Pure oxygen excessively accelerates the metabolic rate, causing the body to essentially burn itself out. It also results in the formation of cellular poisons known as free radicals. The latter greatly disrupt metabolism and can even cause cell death. The free radicals are highly toxic to all cells in the body. Eventually, the excessively high or artificial amounts of oxygen may precipitate organ failure and, thus, premature death. This is why in nature air contains only a small percentage of oxygen. Normally, this is approximately 20%. Thus, air is naturally a mixture of gases, mainly nitrogen and oxygen with a small amount of carbon dioxide. Normally, the carbon dioxide level in the atmosphere is lower than 1%. However, as a result of pollution the levels are continuously rising. Thus, even the fresh air we breathe is inadequate for optimal health, because the body regards any inhaled carbon dioxide as noxious. Carbon monoxide, the gas resulting from automobile emissions, is even more noxious and is, in fact, a lung and tissue poison. High levels of carbon monoxide in inhaled air can quickly lead to death.

J. C. McKendrick, in *Principles of Physiology*, provides a fascinating overview of the function of the lungs. He describes how breathing allows the excretion of carbon in the form of carbon dioxide. This carbon dioxide is produced as a result of normal cellular activities. All living cells, plant and animal, produce it. This gas is found in various organs as well as the blood and lymph. This lymph readily absorbs toxic gases, so it must be continuously decontaminated.

The lymph provides the cells with nutrients, but it is also a respiratory organ, closely tied to every breath. Breathing moves lymph, in other words, the lungs act as a sort of heart for the lymphatic system. Every time we breathe, lymph is pumped. The lymph absorbs oxygen from the lungs and delivers it to the cells, which then dump carbon dioxide back into it. Ultimately, the lymphatics dump the carbon dioxide-rich fluid into the blood so it can be disposed of. In other words, the lungs act to remove the poisonous carbon compounds from the lymph. This is why the lungs are surrounded by lymphatic vessels.

Mouth breathing: a source of illness

Few people realize it, but it is dangerous to breathe through the mouth. The mouth is naturally the passage for food. The lungs are the passage for air. Reversing this is abnormal. William Krohn, M.D., author of *Physiology and Hygiene*, claims mouth breathing is "very harmful." He states that air should always be breathed through the lungs, that is through the nostrils. The lungs and bronchial tubes, he says, are designed to receive air, to condition, moisten, and filter it. The nostrils, acting as the smelling organ, help us sense dangerous odors, toxins, and harmful compounds, which may, as a result, be avoided. With mouth breathing no such warning occurs. Thus, mouth breathing may allow us to breathe unhealthy air continuously, air which we might have sought to avoid had we used our natural nasal sensor system. Dr. Krohn describes that the person who habitually breathes through the mouth may experience a variety of symptoms, while having no clue that it is due to mouth breathing. Symptoms of mouth breathing include dry throat, colds, stuffy sinuses, stuffy nose, runny nose, and even lung disease. In fact, Dr. Krohn explains that the development of lung disease is a certainty as a result of continuous mouth breathing. Incredibly, he claims that colds can be easily prevented by breaking this habit.

The lungs are the main organs of respiration. All other organs, like the nose, trachea, sinuses, and bronchi, are ancillary. The lungs are arranged in a magnificent manner. Miraculously, they have a massive surface area, allowing the greatest possible exposure for air, that is oxygen, absorption.

Respiration is not just to bring in air: it is also to purify the blood. The fluids in our bodies, the blood and lymph, are formed as a result of digestion. In other words what is eaten leads to the creation of the nutritive body fluids. Blood delivers the nutrients from the food to the cells, plus it removes toxins, so they can be excreted. The more toxic is the diet the more toxic will be the various body fluids.

The lymph is also made from food. However, the lymph, which flows towards the heart from the various outer regions of the body, like the limbs, is a waste product. It transports the residues resulting from the degeneration of tissues. Ultimately, the lymph, which resembles a sort of protein-rich cream, is dumped into the bloodstream, and from there it is delivered to the heart.

Like the lymph vessels, the veins carry waste material back toward the heart. The waste laden lymph and venous blood are pumped from the heart into the lungs. Here, these fluids are cleansed and revitalized. Oxygen from the inspired air is the primary cleansing agent.

According to physiology textbooks respiration is defined as the function by which venous blood, that is dark red or bluish-red blood, is converted to arterial blood, that is bright red blood. This, of course, occurs in the lungs and is the result of oxygen. It is also the result of the exhalation of the poisonous carbon dioxide, which is the main agent responsible for the dark color of venous blood. This process of cleansing and detoxifying the blood is absolutely crucial. Any interference with this rapidly results in death, largely because of oxygen deficiency and the accumulation of metabolic poisons. Proper breathing is absolutely crucial in order to prevent such a dangerous circumstance. Any restriction in breathing, as well as the inhalation of poor quality of air, will lead to an increase in metabolic poisons and, therefore, ill health.

Most people fail to breathe properly. They rarely take the time to take deep breaths. Or, they are under an extreme amount of stress and, thus, their breathing is inhibited or constrained. This perpetuates poor health and may lead to actual disease. To become as healthy as possible it is crucial to improve your breathing habits. Take time to take deep breaths. Find out what you are doing that is impeding or restricting your breathing. Improvement in the breathing process will often result in a dramatic enhancement in health.

The importance of deep breathing

Lung disease is often the result of improper breathing practices. It seems rather incredible; however, some people forget to breathe.

Others restrict their breathing because of poor posture. In fact, because of their stress levels they restrict their breathing.

Breathing is an art. It is a form of exercise. Many individuals have conditioned themselves to breathe improperly. Thus, it may be necessary to get a breathing coach or buy books, videos, or tapes, which teach proper breathing exercises. A lack of proper breathing curbs the intake of oxygen, the most necessary of all nutrients. A deficiency of oxygen may cause hundreds of symptoms. This is because, again, oxygen is the most essential of all nutrients. This may explain the rather sudden improvement people experience simply by improving their breathing.

Sleeping: your position affects your health

The Prophet Muhammad was the first to delineate the importance of sleeping positions. He recommended foremost sleeping on the right side. Here is what he said. First, choose the right side for sleeping, and make every attempt to discipline yourself to do so. If you must have an alternative, try the left side. Avoid sleeping on the back. However, the worst position, according to the Prophet, is stomach sleeping.

His recommendations are medically sound. Let us review these recommendations from a scientific/medical point of view: "Sleep on the right side." This makes physiological sense. The heart is tucked next to the rib cage on the left side, its tip pointing downward at an angle towards the back of the rib cage. Sleeping on the left side forces the ribs directly against the heart, impairing its ability to pump blood. This causes the heart to work harder, wearing it out more quickly and increasing the risks for heart failure. The aorta, the major tube guiding blood from the heart to the rest of the body, is also on the left side. By sleeping on the left side, the weight of the body is against it and this partially collaps-es it. This partially impedes the flow of blood to the body. Thus, sleeping on the right side is the ideal position, because it is in con-cert with the laws of gravity. Right-sided sleeping allows the blood to flow freely. Sleeping on the back causes vertebral strain, espe-cially in the lower back. Persistent back sleeping is a major cause of chronic lower back pain. What's more, sleeping on the back creates torque on the lower thoracic and upper lumbar vertebrae. These vertebrae are attached to the diaphragm, the key muscle responsible for breathing. Sleeping on the back greatly strains the diaphragm, making it work exceptionally hard. Back sleeping also compromises the function of the heart. Again, the natural position would be for the heart to lay against the left side of the right lung. Thus, the heart is resting upon soft tissue instead of bone. This allows blood to be pumped without restriction. Thus, sleeping on the right side greatly reduces structural and gravitational stress on the heart and arteries, as is illustrated by the following case history:

> Mr. S. suffered from chronic heart failure, which failed
> to respond to medications. He was placed on a special diet,
> given osteopathic manipulative treatments (to balance the
> spine and release restrictions), and told to sleep only on his
> right side. Within a month he improved dramatically. His
> cardiac condition was ultimately completely resolved.

Stomach sleeping is the most dangerous of all positions. Such a position completely violates the normal physiology of the body. The lungs must expand. Stomach sleeping is essentially sleeping with the full weight of the body upon them. Thus, since the lungs are soft tissues, their expansion is greatly inhibited by fighting against the weight of the body. Obviously, this prevents the lungs from properly functioning. What's more, because of the pressure of the weight of the body against the delicate respiratory tract, stomach sleeping encourages mouth breathing. The fact is stomach sleeping is so dangerous that it may be considered a significant cause of lung and sinus diseases as well as perhaps a cause of premature death.

Every effort should be made to break the stomach sleeping habit. This is precisely what it is: merely a habit. When this is halted, a major improvement in health will result. As an osteopathic physician I observed a number of patients who had damaged their spinal structures, posture, and body conformation, as well as their overall health, through persistent stomach sleeping. Eventually, through a change in position and osteopathic manipulative therapy much of the damage was reversed.

Technique for stopping stomach sleeping

I learned the following technique from one of my old osteopathic professors. Get a pair of old nylons. Within them place two or three tennis balls (if these are unavailable use golf balls). Tie this around the abdomen of the stomach-sleeper, with the balls lying directly around the stomach. Lie on the bed on the right or left side. When the individual rolls over, he or she will experience a rather unpleasant sensation. Note to the assisting spouse: do not allow the culprit to slip this device off during the night. Be vigilant. The only result will be superior health. Any habit is worth breaking for such a price.

Chapter 2

Where Disease Lurks

Air is supposedly healthy, yet, it can be the most dangerous thing on earth. The air may either nourish and sustain us or sicken and poison us. Gases are among the most poisonous substances known. The wrong kinds of gases can kill more quickly than the most deadly oral poison.

Dangerous air, everywhere

The air in virtually every civilized region is contaminated. Certainly, the air in major North American cities is unfit for breathing. In huge cities, such as Los Angeles, Chicago, New York City, San Diego, San Francisco, Atlanta, and Toronto, it is essentially poisonous.

One study determined that people living in Los Angeles suffer tremendous lung damage. In fact, the majority of residents who live in this city for more than ten years suffer from a type of chronic emphysema. This means children living in this region are in essence doomed to suffer permanent lung damage, all the result of environmental contamination.

There are hundreds of pollutants in city air. The majority of these pollutants arise from vehicular exhaust. Industrial exhaust fouls the air with a host of toxins, including mercury, lead, arsenic, cadmium, beryllium, sulfur dioxide, carbon dioxide, carbon monoxide, dioxins, toxic hydrocarbons, and thousands of others. Jet exhaust is an enormous contributor to air pollution. In cities with international airports the air may be so polluted as to be deemed virtually cancerous.

Basement air—unusually dangerous

Avoid basements, especially in strange houses. Go into them only if absolutely necessary. One of the quickest ways to compromise health is to breathe basement air, especially in an individual who is already ill. The exception is basements which have plenty of sunlight or in which fresh air is circulated by opening windows or patio doors. If the basement has no sunlight, then the air may well be deadly. The fact is such basements, devoid of sunlight and ventilation, should have posted at their entrance: Warning: enter at your own risk.

Stagnant basement air is permeated with potentially disease producing germs and noxious gases. The greatest threats are the molds, which thrive in the cold, dark and often moist environment. A great deal of illness could be prevented by simply avoiding entering strange basement environments.

Basements breed disease. The lack of sunlight encourages the growth of a wide range of pathogens, especially molds and fungi. When the lack of sunlight is combined with excessive moisture, the scenario is set for massive mold growth. Merely inhaling this foul air may cause symptoms if not frank illness.

It is important to be aware of how dangerous this air is. This is because millions of individuals develop various symptoms of illness, having no idea it is caused by the air they breathe. What's more, basement air is so dangerous that a few inhalations of contaminated air may lead to a lung or sinus infection. Basement air, filled with mold, poisons and spores, can cause a wide range of symptoms. A partial list includes:

- sinus attacks
- runny nose
- post nasal drip
- sinus pain
- sinus headaches
- pain in the head
- neck pain
- neck stiffness
- rash
- joint pain
- achiness
- flu-like symptoms
- pneumonia
- chest pain
- depression
- agitation
- psychotic behavior
- attention deficit
- itchy skin
- itchy scalp
- cold sensations
- sore throat

This is an incredibly long and varied list of symptoms, all due to the inhalation of poisonous, mold-infested air. This fully illustrates how dangerous the air is in moldy regions. Thus, if you are exposed to such air, the appropriate precautions must be taken to avoid serious illnesses if not outright disease. Even cancer has been associated with mold infestation. A low white count may also be caused by mold poisoning. Molds produce toxins, known descriptively as mycotoxins, which greatly depress the immune system. These toxins are routinely produced as long as the molds actively grow in the body. Obviously, molds have a dire effect upon the immune and respiratory systems, as is illustrated by the following case history:

Mr. C. is a 40 year old with a tendency of developing sinus problems. Recently, his basement was flooded, and a number of books and other items were soaked. The water was cleaned out, but after the flood a noticeable odor developed. He went down to inspect it and detected a foul odor. Soon thereafter he developed severe neck and head pain, the pain in the head being across the occiput (back of the head). He felt cold all over and sluggish. Reasoning that he had developed mold poisoning, he took large amounts of Oreganol (oil of wild oregano) as well as the desiccated spice (Oregacyn). The symptoms quickly dissipated, and he was free of all pain within two hours. He was exceptionally impressed at his rapid improvement, because when he had developed similar "mold" reactions previously, the symptoms lasted for days or weeks.

Chemical pollutants

In North America the inhalation of noxious chemicals is a monumental cause of disability, ill health, and even death. It is also one of the major causes of lung and throat cancer.

The United States is the most chemically polluted region in the world. Tens of thousands of chemicals are used in industry, agriculture, and home use. What's more, industry has never been fully held accountable for the scope of the damages caused. Thus, there is seemingly no curb against their continued pollution of the environment. The exposure to noxious chemicals is a daily event. Long term exposure increases the risks for a variety of respiratory diseases, particularly bronchitis, obstructive lung disease, pneumonia, sinusitis, emphysema, and cancer.

People in the United States suffer a vast degree of diseases due directly to chemical pollution. Millions of people are sickened yearly due to such toxicity. While there are no medical cures, natural medicines offer great hope for reversing much of this toxicity. This is because natural medicines help the body remove toxic chemicals. Plus, natural compounds act as antioxidants, helping to minimize the toxicity of synthetic chemicals. Herbs, spices, vitamins, minerals, enzymes, amino acids, and essential fatty acids all offer healing actions in reversing or minimizing the toxicity of airborne pollutants. The most powerful herbs and spices include sage, rosemary, cumin, coriander, oregano, and cloves. Anti-pollution vitamins include vitamin A, beta carotene, vitamin C, pantothenic acid, and folic acid. Minerals which fight pollution toxicity include magnesium, zinc, and selenium, with the latter being the most important one. However, spice extracts are by far the most powerful and rapidly acting of all detoxification agents. They are potent antioxidants, many times more potent than vitamins and minerals. In some instances they are hundreds of times more potent. Plus, they kill both molds and fungi as well as noxious bacteria. They also assist the lungs in removing harmful chemicals. Humans are at such significant risks currently that mere survival may be dependent upon the regular intake of such substances.

There is little that can be done to reverse the air pollution debacle. For the home environment air purifiers/ionizers may help considerably. However, this illustrates the need to consume protective agents to prevent or reverse lung damage. While the antioxidant and lung-protective powers of certain vitamins are well respected, there are even more powerful substances available. Spice extracts have recently been proven to be the most powerful of all. A recent study (2002) by the USDA, that is the United States Department of Agriculture, found that of all natural antioxidants tested spices were the best. What's more, of all common spices the top was wild oregano. It proved to have some 40 times the antioxidant effect of apples and over five times the action of the well respected antioxidants in blueberries. Another significant finding by the USDA was that the potency of the types of oregano varied greatly, with wild oregano apparently being significantly more potent than the commercial types. Truly wild oregano, as well as other wild herbs and spices, such as sage and rosemary, is so powerful in its antioxidant capacities that it is even superior to synthetic antioxidants such as BHT. This clearly illustrates the value of consuming concentrates of wild spices for reversing or preventing chemically-induced cell or lung damage.

A special type of wild spice antioxidant has become available. Known as OxyOrega™, this is a combination of wild oils of oregano and rosemary. According to Taintu these oils are highly effective in preventing oxidative damage. Here, he describes oregano as a water-phase antioxidant, while rosemary is primarily a fat-phase antioxidant. This means that the components of OxyOrega™ resolve all of the body's critical needs for preserving the health of both watery tissues, such as the blood, lymph, and cellular fluids, as well as fatty tissues, such as the skin membranes, cell membranes, and brain. The fact is OxyOrega™ is so complete in its antioxidant powers that there is little need to take the typical litany of antioxidants. The use of vitamin E and beta carotene, while of some value, pale in insignificance compared to OxyOrega's immense antioxidant activity. Couple this with the fact that many commercial antioxidants are solvent extracted or derived from genetically engineered materials and it is readily understood why taking a pure and unprocessed substance made strictly from wild spices is the ideal choice. Furthermore, OxyOrega is well tolerated by individuals with allergies. Thus, this is the ideal antioxidant for replacing vitamin E in the event of soy or wheat allergy. The fact is OxyOrega contains a plethora of natural vitamin E compounds in the form of spice-derived gamma, beta, and delta tocopherols as well as the rare and difficult to procure tocotrienols. Yet, the key component of such a substance is far from the vitamin E molecules. Rather, it is the potent antioxidants known as phenolics. OxyOrega is rich in carvacrol, rosmarinic acid, and carnosinic acid, which are among the most powerful naturally-occurring antioxidants known. For lung detoxification take ten or more drops under the tongue twice daily. For sudden or serious toxic exposure take ten or more drops under the tongue every few minutes until exposure toxicity has been neutralized.

Chapter 3

Germs, Germs, Everywhere

The air that is breathed may seem pure or clean. However, incredibly, it is never sterile. Usually, it is teeming with germs. Yet, germs infect the lungs from sources besides the air. This is because germs in food and water may also infect them.

Bacteria are everywhere

In every breath of air there are germs. Bacteria are regarded as the primary lung pathogens. This creates a great deal of fear, because everyone knows that bacteria are potential killers. However, incredibly, with the exception of tuberculosis, viruses and molds are the main cause of respiratory infections. While less fatal than bacteria they are a major cause of chronic respiratory conditions that defy diagnosis and resist conventional therapies. Yet, bacteria cause a significant amount of lung or respiratory disorders, and this is particularly true of hospitalized and/or post-surgical patients. They are also a primary cause of respiratory infections in nursing home occupants.

With lung bacterial infections the consequences can be severe. If untreated, fatality may rapidly result. Such infections are usually manifested by sudden onset of high fever plus chills.

There is usually a painful cough plus purulent or green- or yellow-colored sputum. Thus, the development of sudden and severe lung infection in a hospitalized or nursing home patient must be regarded as bacterial until proven otherwise.

The role of parasites

A parasite is an organism that cannot live on its own. It must derive its food, nutrition, and housing from its host. In animals parasitic infection is common and is virtually normal. As described by Hanna Kroeger in her book, *Parasites: The Enemy Within*, humans may house as many as 100 types. According to Kroeger the danger is that most Americans regard parasitic diseases as a problem of Third World or tropical countries. They fail to understand that currently parasitic infections are an American epidemic and that tens of millions of individuals are afflicted. Certain investigators regard parasitic infection now to be the norm. In other words, they believe the majority of North Americans suffer from some degree of infestation.

Parasites are a major cause of lung disease. The lungs are a type of filter, and parasites may be trapped there from the blood. Plus, lung tissue is rich in nutrients, and parasites tend to lodge in nutrient-rich tissue. The lungs are rich in red blood: parasites feed off of it.

Doctors rarely diagnose parasitic lung disease. This is mainly because they fail to consider it as a serious possibility. For instance, an entire book, *Introduction to Respiratory Diseases*, published by the National Tuberculosis and Respiratory Disease Association, fails to mention parasites. Thus, there is a lack of education, as well as awareness, for doctors regarding the importance of these noxious germs in causing acute and chronic lung disorders. The poor rate of diagnosis is also because there are few if any tests that can accurately confirm the presence of these organisms within the lungs. It is also because, immediately, physicians consider any severe case of lung infection as bacterial. Yet, globally, parasitic infections cause a far greater number of acute lung infections than even viruses. What's more, they are a significant cause of chronic lung disease. Parasites hide deep within lung tissue and rarely cause any obvious lung signs. In fact, the infection becomes visibly evident only when it is chronic, severe, and massive. What's more, acute parasitic infection is even more rarely diagnosed, largely because doctors fail to consider it. The symptoms mimic more commonly considered infections, including bacterial or viral pneumonia. In fact, when this infection does strike, it is usually diagnosed as the flu or pneumonia. Yet, if a careful history were taken, there would be a higher degree of suspicion and, therefore, a more rapid resolution of symptoms.

If a high level of suspicion became the mainstay, parasitic lung infection would be more commonly discovered. The typical history is as follows: the onset of a rather sudden, severe case of respiratory distress, that is coughing, chest pain, fever, chills, sweating, aches/malaise, combined with the potential exposure to contaminated food or water. A sudden bout of pneumonia in an individual who rarely develops it is another warning. Traveling overseas, while eating uncooked food or drinking various non-sterile beverages, increases the risks and begs the diagnosis. The fact is the individual who develops a severe lung infection while traveling overseas must be considered suffering from lung parasites until proven otherwise.

Fungal infections

This is perhaps the most under-diagnosed of all lung infections. The majority of doctors are aware of it. Yet, often they fail to respect its seriousness or how common it truly is. In an individual with a chronic lung condition that fails to respond to traditional treatment fungal infestation should be seriously considered as the culprit.

Medical texts describe lung fungal infections as "exceedingly common." Exposure to the cause of these infections, that is mold spores, is nearly continuous, especially in warm and/or damp climates. Through the air we breathe these spores readily enter the respiratory tract, lodging in the lungs. They may not immediately cause outright disease, yet they must always be regarded as a foreign irritant. Under certain circumstances, such as stress, drug therapy, or a weakened immune system, they can grow in a fulminant fashion, causing severe respiratory symptoms. A course or two of antibiotics may provoke such an infection. This is because by destroying the inhibitory, healthy bacteria and, thus, altering immunity they encourage the growth of molds and fungi. A wide range of diseases may be caused by mold/fungal infection of the lungs. A partial list includes asthma, chronic or acute bronchitis, pneumonia, sinusitis, earaches, rhinitis, pleurisy, sinus headaches, and pharyngitis.

Molds and fungi readily enter the lungs. To some degree they are filtered by the nose and sinuses. However, mold spores are relatively small and, thus can penetrate deep into the lungs. What's more, if the molds or yeasts infect the sinuses, contaminated secretions may drip into the lungs, infecting them as well.

In contrast to parasites there are a number of medical tests which can aid in determining the existence of lung fungus. The number of fungi which may infect the respiratory tract are legion and include aspergillus, penicillium, histoplasma, coccidiodes, cryptococcus, nocardia, blastomyces, and actinomyces. Many of these fungi are regional, for instance, coccidiodes is a desert fungus and blastomyces is a river valley fungus. Individuals who visit regions where these fungi are endemic are highly vulnerable to developing the disease, because they have no immunity against it. The fact is the people who live there locally may have the infection chronically and not even be aware of it.

Mold in homes

If you suddenly develop a health problem, particularly lung and/or sinus disorders, check for mold in your house. Mold gets into the home in several ways. Moist indoor environments, such as saunas, pool rooms, bathrooms, and damp basements, breed it. Mold spores are constantly circulating in the air and may enter through any opening. However, usually they are residents of closed spaces and are not contaminants from outdoors. Symptoms of mold intoxication may vary greatly. A few of the more common symptoms include:

- Joint pain
- Sinus attacks
- Watery eyes
- Itchy eyes
- Itchy nose

- Attacks of sneezing
- Runny nose
- Headaches
- Pain behind the eye
- Chest pain

- Shortness of breath
- Spastic muscles
- Neck pain
- Spinal stiffness
- Chronic ear infection
- Sudden awakening at night
- Attention deficit
- Forgetfulness
- Anger/frustration
- Confusion
- Lowered energy
- Nausea
- Cough
- Hives
- Scratchy throat
- Exhaustion
- Inability to focus on work
- Bleeding from the lungs (coughing up blood)
- Wheezing
- Loss of bladder control
- Dizziness
- Weakness
- Insomnia
- Poor concentration
- Mood swings
- Psychotic tendencies
- Irritability
- Apathy
- Bloody nose
- Vomiting
- Allergic reactions
- Sore throat
- Hay fever-like symptoms
- Vague abdominal pain
- Spots on the lungs (visible by X ray)

The role of food allergies

Allergies play an enormous role in lung and respiratory problems. In fact, in many instances they may play the predominant role.

Many diseases which are presumed to be infectious may, in fact, be due mainly to food allergies. For instance, I used to be a bronchitis sufferer. Every fall or winter I would get a severe case, which would last for as long as two months. I might endure several episodes per year. Then I learned of the importance of food allergies. Through a sophisticated blood test I discovered my allergenic foods. When I removed those foods from my diet, which included wheat, rye, celery, asparagus, butter, cheddar cheese, perch, baker's yeast, and Swiss cheese, the bronchitis disappeared, never again to return.

The bizarre issue is that the aforementioned foods are technically wholesome. Yet, even seemingly healthy foods can be toxic, that is if you are allergic to them. This toxicity damages the immune system, leaving the body vulnerable to the development of various infections as well as diseases. Thus, the continuous intake of allergenic foods is a major cause of chronic disease.

Allergenic foods have a major impact upon the function and health of the lungs. They cause a significant degree of toxicity, perhaps more so than even airborne allergens. The toxic aspects of such foods directly poison the immune system. This directly impacts the function of the lungs causing a wide range of conditions, including asthma, bronchitis, sinusitis, ear infections, rhinitis, and even pneumonia.

Foods contain hundreds of chemicals in the form of various unique molecules, proteins, sugars, and fats. In other words, they are rather complex substances. Certain of these molecules are known to evoke allergic responses. This is one reason certain natural foods may cause severe reactions. Incredibly, it is possible that something as natural as broccoli or asparagus could cause severe or chronic allergic reactions. Today, this is complicated by the fact that modern foods are heavily processed. This processing renders them more likely to cause allergic toxicity. Plus, they contain added chemicals. These chemicals are aberrant, that is they are synthetic and unknown to nature. Thus, the immune system usually recognizes them as foreign, that is it regards them as toxic. Genetic engineering complicates this, since it increases the types of aberrant chemicals in the foods. As a result the immune cells attack the chemicals and/or the food, setting the stage for allergic intolerance. Thus, the body recognizes the food as a toxin, because it is infiltrated with synthetic, dangerous chemicals.

Food intolerance is a major cause of respiratory disorders. Incredibly, ear infections, colds, flu-like symptoms, sore throats, tonsillitis, asthma, sinus, and bronchial conditions may all be primarily due to food allergies. Thus, food allergy reactions are the great mimicker. Could a sore throat be caused by food allergies? Indeed, I have seen dozens of cases where the continual consumption of noxious or allergenic foods leads to terrible sore throats. Antibiotics are taken in an attempt to quell the pain and supposed infection. However, they are ineffective. In fact, they may perpetuate the illness. This is because antibiotics depress immunity, increasing the likelihood for allergic intolerance. Plus, this approach fails to take into account the fact that toxic foods depress the immune system, and, thus, the germ infections are merely secondary. In other words, the germs are merely opportunists. Even strep throat may have its origin from food allergy, because these allergic reactions deplete the immune reserve, making the throat vulnerable to bacterial invasion.

The majority of people, especially those with chronic diseases, are allergic to certain foods. There is great variance in people regarding the specific toxic foods. Just why each individual has his/her own pattern of allergenic foods is largely unknown. Heredity may play a role, as does the individual's dietary habits. Regarding the latter simply consuming certain foods to an excess may result in allergy. In fact, this is one of the most common causes of food allergies. Environmental toxins are another major cause. The toxins enter the food supply and become concentrated in certain foods. As mentioned previously when the foods are eaten, the body recognizes them as poisonous and, thus, allergic intolerance develops.

Food allergies can result in dozens of respiratory symptoms. A partial list includes:

• Runny nose	• Itchy eyes
• Itchy nose	• Plugged sinuses
• Sinus infections	• Sinus headaches
• Wheezing	• Asthma attacks
• Bronchitis	• Post nasal drip
• Earaches	• Ear discharge
• Fever/chills	• Chronic cough
• Hoarseness	• Laryngitis
• Itchy ears	• Shortness of breath
• Sore throat	• Sneezing spells
• Pneumonia	• Chest pain

From this list it becomes apparent that a number of lung diseases may be caused at least in part by food intolerances. Thus, it is crucial to discover the exact food intolerances in order to enhance the healing processes. Removing the food toxicities significantly aids in the cure. This is an issue of major importance. By avoiding the toxic food the immune system is relieved of a significant burden, and, or as a result, the health improves dramatically.

The majority of food allergy tests, including the well-known scratch test, which is used by the majority of allergy specialists, are inaccurate. The scratch test is notorious for its poor accuracy for foods, with a precision of less than 30%. Rast testing is even worse, with an accuracy of only 5-10%. The fact is the results of the majority of food allergy tests may prove misleading. A specialized, highly accurate food allergy test is available. Known as the Food Intolerance Test, it is a blood test requiring merely a single tube of blood. It boasts an accuracy of approximately 70% or better. The blood is processed and then carefully analyzed under a special microscope. Over 205 foods and food additives are carefully screened.

The test is based upon a principle of immunology regarding how toxins interact with the actual blood cells. Technicians view toxic reactions of food extracts against three types of cells: red blood cells, platelets, and white blood cells. The toxic reactions are measured as mild, moderate, and severe, and this is scored on the food chart as respectively 1, 2, or 3. A score of three indicates a severe intolerance, and such foods must be avoided strictly. Ideally, all allergenic foods, whether 1, 2, or 3, should be avoided for at least 90 days. Afterwards, each food may be re-introduced into the diet, starting with those scoring 1, but consumed no more than once every five days. When re-introducing such foods, do eat them in small quantities. However, if such foods cause noticeable reactions, they should be avoided indefinitely.

Currently, the Food Intolerance Test is only performed at one facility. It is a research-quality test and, therefore, is not available through standard medical laboratories. The cost is approximately $2.00 per food, which is a tremendous value considering the amount of information that is generated. Other testing may cost as much as $12.00 per food, while being less accurate. The total cost for some 205 foods is $400.00.

To perform this test a special test tube with the appropriate blood preservative is required. Your doctor can order this test for you. Or, the appropriate lab can draw the blood and send it. The tube must be sent either to your doctor's office or the lab. Then, the technician will draw your blood and send it in. For more information contact:

Food Intolerance Test
1701 Golf Rd Suite 606 Tower 2
Rolling Meadows, IL 60008
(800) 295-3737

While in many individuals one test may be sufficient, ideally, it may be appropriate to repeat the test every year. Strict avoidance of allergenic foods may result in the reversal of many of the allergies. However, there may be certain substances or foods in which the individual is allergic that should be avoided permanently, such as food additives, as is illustrated by the following case history:

Mr. J. had a history of severe sinus attacks. His sinuses would become completely plugged, causing pain and, occasionally, sinus headaches. Food intolerance testing proved he was allergic to several foods, particularly butter and cheese. Plus, he was allergic to a number of food additives, including aspartame (i.e. NutraSweet). Removing the NutraSweet alone led to a significant improvement, and his sinus condition disappeared within a month.

The power of spice extracts: nature's germ killers

Spice extracts have proven germ-killing powers. They don't discriminate: they kill virtually every pathogen, that is harmful germ. A number of spices have been studied for their germ killing powers. Chief of these is oil of wild oregano. Other extracts which kill a wide range of germs include oils of cinnamon, clove, allspice, garlic, onion, cumin, myrtle, bay leaf, sage, and thyme.

The oils from certain strains of wild oregano are potent germicides, capable of killing a wide range of germs. The use of only wild oregano oil is crucial, since farm-raised oregano is far weaker. Avoid all farm-raised types.

Oil of wild oregano is capable of killing all known germs. The exception is anthrax, which, while initially killed by the oregano oil, tends to regrow. However, no other germ has been proven to resist it. Even so, evidence exists that the most potent approach is to combine a number of antiseptic spices. This creates an additive, that is synergistic, action, which is invaluable for the natural treatment of difficult-to-kill germs. Recent research at major reference labs indicates that a combination of wild spice extracts, including the P73 oregano, is more aggressive in destroying anthrax than oil of oregano alone. The fact is the oil of oregano alone failed to achieve a complete kill. Yet, a combination of spice oils destroyed this germ. These spice extracts are, in fact, the components of Oregacyn.

Oregacyn is a multi-spice extract made from wild and mountain-grown spices and herbs. It offers the synergy, that is the additive action, of numerous antiseptic spices. Yet, what is of particular importance is that spice extracts possess additional medicinal properties. They are potent antioxidants, far more powerful than mere vitamins and minerals. They are also anti-histaminic, meaning they combat allergies. Many spice extracts exert beneficial actions on the lungs, for instance, helping to thin or dry excessive mucous. Potent spice extracts, such as those in Oregacyn, also exhibit anti-pain properties. This is largely due to the incredible quantity of simple phenols they contain.

Oregacyn is a special blend of multiple spices, including extracts of wild oregano (the researched P73 blend), wild sage, and wild, mountain-grown cumin. The cumin in Oregacyn is 100% wild. Research at major reference labs has proven that wild cumin is over three times more powerful than the commercial or farm-raised types. The oils are extracted and then powdered through a proprietary process that maintains, in fact, enhances potency. Oregacyn is perhaps the most potent nutritional supplement available. Plus, it is edible, and, thus, is ideal for all ages. Use it for immune support when the body needs strengthening against stress, germs, chronic pain, or other immune weaknesses. Yet, its greatest power is due to one fact: it kills germs outright. Plus, Oregacyn, being an edible multiple-spice extract, has a natural, spicy taste. Open the capsule and add it to soup, stir fry, cheese dip, or meat dishes. It is still useful when cooked, but, ideally, take it in the capsule as needed, one or more capsules daily. For tough situations take 2 or more capsules twice daily.

Chapter 4

Respiratory Illnesses and Their Natural Cures

In North America respiratory conditions account for a greater number of diseases than any other category. Today, illnesses affecting the respiratory organs, such as the lungs, sinuses, ear canals, throat, etc., are the main causes of sickness. It is well known that respiratory illnesses are the number one cause of doctors' visits. Think about it. When you visit a doctor, what is it usually for? Isn't it usually a sore throat, tonsillitis, laryngitis, flu, cold, sinus attack, earache, etc.? Everyone knows how much trepidation there is during cold and flu season. The fact is these illnesses can strike at anytime. What's more, the hospitals and doctors' offices are often overwhelmed by the sickened. Put simply, many people fear the thought of becoming seriously ill from winter or respiratory illnesses. This is rightfully so. Such illnesses can prove deadly.

Medical therapy for respiratory illnesses is lacking. Few if any cures are offered. Asthma is an excellent example. While there are numerous drugs available, as well as specialized types of respiratory therapies, the results are often poor. In fact, since the 1930s there has been a 400% rise in the death rate. The major difference is that during that era few if any pharmaceutical drugs were available.

Numerous scientific studies delineate the fact that the current treatment for asthma increases the risks for complications. It also increases the risks for death. Unfortunately, regarding medical therapy today the same can be said for various lung infections such as pneumonia and bronchitis. Drugs which were once highly effective are now rendered useless, largely because of their overuse. Not only are the antibiotics virtually impotent, but they may often accelerate germ growth. Incredibly, it has been determined that certain bacteria actually use certain antibiotics as fuel. They alter the antibiotic molecule and feast upon it. In hospitals today resistant bacteria routinely infect the lungs and bronchial tubes. What's more, they are virtually impossible to kill, that is except with natural medicines. One study at Georgetown University showed that spice extracts, notably oil of wild oregano, destroyed drug-resistant staph. The researchers, using a blend of wild oregano oils known as P73, were able to destroy the staph, even within tissue. After 30 days not a trace of this toxic bacteria could be found. Drug-resistant staph is a primary cause of illness, as well as death, in hospitalized patients. In one study in laboratory animals the oregano oil blend was more effective than the antibiotic Vancomycin, the latter usually being regarded as a last resort. These incredible results illustrate the immense potential of natural compounds in the treatment of infectious disease. In fact, such compounds will be the cures of the future.

There are three major categories of respiratory illnesses: the common everyday illnesses, such as colds, flu, and earache, which are rarely serious, the potentially serious diseases, such as bronchitis, asthma, and pneumonia, which may be fatal, and the obscure illnesses, such as asbestosis and sarcoidosis, which are frequently fatal. Cancer could be regarded as perhaps a fourth category, as there are dozens of types of respiratory cancers. What follows is a rather comprehensive list of the most common respiratory diseases and their natural, dietary, nutritional, and herbal cures.

Actinomycosis

This, as the name indicates (i.e. "mycosis"), is a type of fungus. This fungus readily grows in the respiratory system and may invade the lymph glands, especially the glands under the jaw. It is contracted as a result of exposure to grain, like grain dust. The dust can be infective, because this organism lives on raw grain. Thus, this disease commonly develops in farmers. It may also develop in individuals who work with flour, like workers in granaries, flour mills, or bakeries. This is because the fungus may hide on flour dust and, thus, may be inhaled.

Actinomycosis is highly invasive, although it normally only invades the tissues of individuals with weakened constitutions. It most commonly attacks the glands under the jaw and may even invade the jawbone, causing a type of osteomyelitis (bone sepsis). In many individuals this germ is an oral resident, but is not necessarily infective. Invasive dentistry may spread it, causing active infection. The teeth are a major reservoir for this germ. An infected tooth may continuously seed this organism into the bloodstream and/or tissues, causing chronic illness. The germ may also attack the tongue and throat. The lungs are readily infected, and the resulting symptoms may mimic tuberculosis. Here, it may hide, growing slowly for years. It may ultimately destroy the lungs, leading to chronic bronchitis and/or emphysema. The lung infection may be difficult to eradicate, and there are no drugs to treat this condition. However, spice extracts destroy this fungus. Thus, the regular intake of antiseptic spice oils may prove lifesaving.

This infection may be readily prevented. Precautions should be taken by both farmers and individuals who process/handle raw grain. If you are in this category, consider wearing a mask during potential exposure. Antifungal essential oils, such as oil of lavender, oil of wild rosemary, and oil of wild oregano, should be administered. They may be taken orally or administered into the air through atomizers or vaporizers. If wearing a mask, saturate a portion of it with a few drops of oil of wild oregano (Oreganol P73) and/or wild lavender oil. Or, spray Germ-a-Clenz in the involved area to decontaminate it. Rapid and thorough destruction of this germ is mandatory. As a means of prevention take a capsule or two of Oregacyn on a daily basis. Actinomycosis is a potentially fatal disease.

Treatment protocol

Take a potent natural antiseptic, such as Oregacyn, one or more capsules twice daily. For tough cases increase the dose, for instance, three capsules three times daily with meals. Also, use oil of wild Oreganol for oral cleansing. Add a drop or two to toothpaste or use it directly on the toothbrush. Rub a drop or two on the teeth and gums at night. Also, for active infection take five to ten drops under the tongue two or more times daily. Use the Germ-a-Clenz as an environmental decontaminant.

Be consistent: this is a difficult organism to eradicate. Stay on this program for at least 60 days. Take also a healthy bacteria supplement, such as Health-Bac, a large dose at night before bedtime. If you are exposed to grain or grain dust, take appropriate precautions like wearing a mask or maintaining proper ventilation. Wash the hands frequently. Add a few drops of oil of wild oregano to pump soaps.

Anthrax

For thousands of years anthrax has been known as a disease of animals, particularly herbivores. The anthrax bacteria, Bacillus anthracis, thrives in moist soil. Thus, it may contaminate grass and hay. Animals become infected by eating contaminated grass/hay or by inhaling the spores. Sheep, goats, horses, and cows are particularly susceptible to it. If the exposure is significant, it may infect all their organs, causing death.

People may occasionally contract anthrax by direct exposure with animals. Animal caretakers may develop it, although it is exceptionally rare. It may be contracted from an infected animal, soil, or objects that were contaminated with animal wastes, or residues in animal products, like wool or hides. The fact is during the early 1900s anthrax was known as Wool-sorter's disease. While less common, as described in the 1970s publication, *Family Health Guide*, human to human transmission may occur. This is in contrast to the current claim, which is that it is not contagious. Yet, Dr. Greer's *A Physician in the House* describes that animals which die from this disease "reek with contagion." What's more, he describes how those who handle infected tissues "are extremely liable to be poisoned...and even flies from such animals may convey (it) to human beings." Yet, admittedly, today such a mode of spread would be rare.

Currently, the major concern surrounds anthrax spores. The bacteria that causes anthrax belongs to a category of germs known as spore-forming bacteria. The spore is a dormant form, meaning it may readily cause infection at a later date. According to *Jordan's General Bacteriology* the anthrax spore is one of the most resistant, that is tough-to-kill, of all bacterial forms. This is largely because the spore is coated with a highly resistant shell. The typical germicides are rather impotent against it. For instance, mercuric chloride, an outright poison, fails to kill it even after an hour long exposure, whereas this germicide kills virtually every other germ. However, heat and steam can kill it, although it takes ten minutes to do so.

There are four forms of anthrax. The most serious is the inhalation variety, which kills the majority of its victims. This is caused by the direct inhalation of anthrax spores. Once inhaled, the spores, which are sort of a bacterial seed, develop rapidly within the lungs. Within minutes or at the maximum a few hours the lungs are flooded with bacteria, which invade the entire system. Ultimately, the bacteria overgrow in such vast numbers that they create a mechanical plug, suffocating the breathing mechanism. Plus, the anthrax bacteria produce potent toxins, which cause the body to go into shock. When anthrax enters any biological fluid, as found in the lungs or blood, it reproduces in vast numbers, causing grave danger. Billions of such germs may grow in a matter of hours. Microbiological texts describe the observance of "enormous multiplication." These texts describe how the capillaries, the tiny blood vessels found in the internal organs, are "gorged" with these very large bacteria. The gastrointestinal type, which is more rare, is also highly fatal. It is usually caused by eating anthrax-contaminated meat or drinking contaminated milk. Also, there is the skin type, which is characterized by the development of circular skin lesions at the site of infection. With this type, systemic symptoms, like headache, nausea, and vomiting, may also develop. The malignant skin type may also be manifested by swelling of the tissues just below the skin, that is the subcutaneous tissues. This may result in sloughing of the skin: even gangrene.

Dr. Greer describes the transmission of cutaneous anthrax: "Wherever (it) enters the system, usually at some abraded point on the skin, a malignant pustule is formed on the fourth day after inoculation, and quickly enlarges and ulcerates and looks malignant...the nearest glands become enlarged. There is general fever and great prostration, which may be followed by collapse and death in four or five days." Interestingly, Dr. Greer described a possible cure. If the lesion was treated as soon as it developed with cautery, the progression could be halted. A common medical procedure, cautery is the use of heat directed at the skin through a hot iron or electrified probe. Perhaps this should be again investigated in the local treatment of anthrax lesions. Yet, there are less painful and more safe means of cautery: the application of phenolic extracts. Plant phenols exert a sort of "chemical cauterization" action. This action is potent, safe, and effective. While medical treatment for this condition is advised, the application of natural phenol-rich extracts, such as the oils of cinnamon and wild oregano, would be an invaluable adjunct for the reversal of pustular microbial lesions. A multiple spice extract, such as oil of Oregacyn, would be even superior, since anthrax is exceptionally difficult to kill.

Even if the anthrax bacteria are killed, there is another concern: the anthrax toxin. Antibiotics fail to disable it, and, thus, the toxin may induce further organ damage, perhaps death. This is why it is crucial to rely upon the powers of natural cures. Certain herbs contain antitoxins. Spice extracts are among the most potent antitoxins known. Turkish investigators proved that oil of wild oregano neutralized aflatoxin, one of the most dangerous biological toxins known. Thus, it is the ideal antidote in the event of exposure to a biological toxin. The fact is oil of wild Oreganol is capable of immediately neutralizing this toxin.

According to certain departments at the federal government natural cures for anthrax are regarded as ineffective. The claim is that there is a lack of proof. Yet, there is no scientific proof that drugs cure it. True, antibiotics could prove lifesaving. However, there are no drugs capable of neutralizing anthrax toxin. What's more, drug resistance of anthrax to antibiotics is increasing. Thus, the approach should be to discover natural compounds that could act as antidotes to the toxin, while killing the bacteria. The fact is any agent that could be of value should be explored, that is if the objective is to protect the sanctity of human life.

The "lack of proof" statement is itself false. The fact is a number of studies have shown that anthrax may be killed with certain natural compounds, particularly spice oils. Egyptian researchers found that oils of cinnamon and cumin, both of which are found in Oregacyn, outright destroyed anthrax bacteria. This was confirmed by an EPA-registered lab, which determined that the combination of oils used in Oregacyn were capable in massive amounts of destroying this bacteria's sister germ, *Bacillus subtilus*. Other investigators have determined that Bacillus subtilus is highly susceptible to oils of oregano, garlic, and thyme. The fact is natural compounds play a significant role in protecting the body from infection. Furthermore, in the early 1900s, when anthrax was more common in America, medical doctors used a synthetic version of the active ingredient of spice extracts, that is phenol. They gave it orally, two drops twice daily, finding it "somewhat successful." According to *Beyond Antibiotics* the natural phenols of oregano are 21 times more potent than synthetic phenols. Interestingly, in the early 1900s synthetic phenol, that is carbolic acid, was relied upon for gastrointestinal anthrax.

While the claim that spice extracts are the cure for anthrax cannot be made, further research may determine that such compounds are even more potent than the synthetics. In summary, regarding anthrax the following are some of the most critical issues:

a) it usually presents with symptoms that in a general way mimic the flu

b) facial and nasal symptoms, such as runny nose, stuffy nose, cough, watery eyes, and sore throat, probably indicate a virus, not anthrax

c) early symptoms of the inhalation variety often include deep pain in the front of the chest.

d) early signs of the skin form of anthrax are a red spot on the skin followed by a vesicle, which is usually painless and which has a center, with dead cells.

e) the diagnosis requires a variety of medical tests plus a high level of suspicion. Nasal swabs only tell the degree of inhalation of spores.

Treatment protocol

The medical treatment for anthrax is the antibiotic, Cipro. It is mandatory to bolster the immune system in this disease. Take a phenolic-based multi-spice extract, such as Oregacyn, two or more capsules three times daily. For severe infection increase the dose to up to five capsules every hour. Be sure to take such a dose with food. In the event of dire need take two or more capsules every hour. Also, take Super Strength Oreganol, about ten or more drops every hour. On a daily basis drink also the juice of three yellow onions. The taste may be disguised with parsley juice. This onion juice therapy, while difficult, is one of the most powerful, lifesaving anthrax treatments known. It may be relied upon to induce a rapid cure. Also, for lung toxicity rub Respira Clenz on the chest as often as needed. Plus, take 20 or more drops of Respira Clenz three times daily. For skin lesions rub with Super Strength oil of oregano as often as needed. Top with a poultice of raw honey. For skin pustules apply a poultice of oil of wild oregano in raw honey. Add 20 drops of Oregano in 1/4 cup honey. Apply as needed daily until lesions are eradicated.

Asbestos contamination (Asbestosis)

Asbestos is a fibrous compound made from minerals, mainly magnesium and silica (magnesium silicate). It is of importance, because fibers of this dangerous material easily become airborne. Inhalation of the fibers occurs mainly in factory workers. In the earlier part of the 20th century this occurred more commonly, since the dangers of asbestos fibers were largely unknown. However, today individuals who work with asbestos are carefully protected by masks and a host of strict regulations.

Usually, it takes several years of exposure to create the disease. The fibers are deposited in the bronchiole tubes. There, they stimulate scar tissue formation. The scars eventually completely consume the lungs, leading to severe breathing difficulty and, ultimately, respiratory collapse and death.

Asbestos poisoning is a significant cause of death and disability. The *Chicago Tribune*, September 2001, reported the degree of human misery it can cause. An entire town, Libby, Montana, is suffering from the poisoning. Mining created dust, which residents inhaled. Some 200 people have died and thousands of others are chronically ill. This is only a small measure of the debacle. In Libby it is estimated that the entire town is at risk. This means that thousands of people may suffer permanent lung damage as a result of such pollution. Despite extensive precautions tens of thousands of North Americans suffer from it. In the year 2000 alone work-related claims for asbestos exposure numbered 50,000. Medical costs, as well as costs for cleanup, number in the tens of billions. In Libby, Montana, the crisis is so dire that Chris Weis of the EPA called it "the most severe residential exposure to a hazardous material this country has ever seen." Thus, it is no surprise that death rates from asbestosis in this town are up to 60 times greater than the national average. These people are suffering unmercifully, an agony that was largely preventable. Incredibly, up to 30% of the town members are victims of the disease. Yet, despite the fact that the risks were known, nothing was done by the government. The people were left uninformed and unprotected. Only after the residents themselves filed a series of lawsuits did the degree of the danger become exposed. The fact is the government became involved only after the lawsuits were filed.

News reports of the lawsuits reached the EPA's Paul Peronard, who found the reports difficult to believe. Yet, when he investigated it, he found that the suffering was beyond comprehension. In fact, the Libby experience utterly demolished the old theories about asbestosis, that is that it took prolonged regular exposure, requiring decades to develop. Rather, people became sick far more quickly than what was previously understood: in just a few years or less. Direct exposure was unnecessary. Just living in the area was enough risk. In this debacle it is expected that thousands of individuals will live in utter misery, dying a slow, miserable death. The fact is they are suffocating to death.

To cure this condition it is necessary to dissolve the asbestos fibers. Yet, incredibly, the condition is far from hopeless. Nature can again come to the rescue. This may be accomplished by essential oil therapy. Essential oils are solvents, and, thus, they help dissolve and decompose particulate matter. Also, they act as lymphatic stimulants, that is they aid in the flow of lymph, and it is the lymphatic ducts which become plugged in asbestosis. Thus, the regular intake of edible essential oils can prove lifesaving in this condition. The oils which are particularly valuable include oils of wild oregano, rosemary, lavender, neroli, sage, cloves, and juniper. The fact is by dissolving organic particulate matter these oils greatly assist lung function. Particulate matter in the lungs significantly interferes with the function of these organs. In many instances, even a relatively tiny amount of inhaled particles can create disease.

Recently, an Italian study provided definitive proof of the immense value of this treatment. The study found that essential oils turn asbestos fibers into harmless polymers. Once this occurs the asbestos can be readily decontaminated. Unlike the fibers, the polymers are inert. Thus, they fail to induce scarring. This means that the fatal aspects of this mineral can be neutralized precisely with natural compounds. Plus, once they are acted upon by these oils the fibers may be digested by the immune system and, therefore, rendered harmless. Oil of wild oregano is one of the most aggressive of these de-polymerizing oils.

Treatment protocol

As mentioned in ancient holy texts, including the Bible, wild oregano is regarded as a "cleansing" herb. It is described in the Bible as a "purge." Research documents this precise function. A study at Georgetown University shows that when tissues are infected with both yeasts and bacteria, oil of wild oregano, in this study using the Oreganol P73, purges the tissues of all traces of germs. No other type of oregano oil was proven effective. Only Oreganol was proven clinically effective. In other words, the Oreganol, which is 100% wild, destroyed the germs so thoroughly that they could no longer be found, nor could they be cultured. The fact is every last trace of the invasive germ was destroyed. In chronic lung conditions, including asbestosis, lung infections may kill. Thus, oil of wild oregano may prove lifesaving.

Hot herbs and spices enhance blood flow, aiding in the removal of toxins. Extracts of certain spices, particularly wild oregano, clove, and thyme, offer significant solvent actions. The solvent powers of oil of wild oregano are immense. This oil can rapidly dissolve asbestos deposits, preventing further lung damage and even curing the condition. To correct this condition take edible oil of wild Oreganol, five or more drops under the tongue several times daily. For difficult cases use the Super Strength oil of Oreganol, five to ten drops under the tongue several times daily. Take also the crude wild oregano, that is Oregamax, two or more capsules twice daily. Other oils which aid in the healing of lung tissue and the removal of contaminants include oils of rosemary, lavender, juniper, cloves, and sage. Make a tea from cinnamon sticks and cloves. Add wild oregano honey and drink two or three cups daily. This type of honey contains natural antiseptics derived from the wild oregano plants. It is only available via mail order: call 1-800-243-5242. Certain vitamins and minerals aid in the removal of asbestos. These vitamins and minerals include beta carotene, vitamin E, vitamin C, selenium, and zinc. Take about 25,000 I.U. of beta carotene daily along with 400 I.U. of vitamin E. Take also a crude natural vitamin C supplement, such as Flavin-C, 3 capsules twice daily. Also, on a daily basis take selenium, 600 mcg and zinc, 75 mg.

Asthma

This disease is represented as sudden attacks of shortness of breath. There are numerous illnesses which may cause these attacks, but not all of them are truly asthmatic. For instance, a severe case of pneumonia may result in shortness of breath, as can a heart attack or congestive heart failure. In fact, in certain instances a heart attack may present as an attack of asthma.

Bronchial asthma is the true type. It afflicts over ten million North Americans. The disease occurs most frequently in children and teenagers, with males being the primary victims.

It is well known that asthmatics react to substances in the air. The dander of animals (i.e. animal dandruff) readily provokes it. Dander or dandruff may contain mold toxins, as well as mite toxins, and these are the likely culprits.

It has been known for decades that asthma has a major allergic component. Yet, it has also been known that infection is a significant cause. Research indicates that of all infectious agents molds and fungi are the primary culprits.

In children asthma often presents with a recurring cough for which a cause cannot be found. Yet, a recurring or persistent cough is a major symptom of disguised infection, particularly fungal or yeast infection. If the cough is not properly diagnosed and treatment offered, the infection would likely worsen, leading to intractable disease.

As early as the 1950s physicians knew that allergic reactions to molds, as well as systemic mold infections, played a critical role in the genesis of asthma. According to Morris Fishbein, M. D., editor of the *Medical and Health Encyclopedia*, in asthma mold sensitivity, as well as outright infection by molds/fungi, plays a "very important role." Furthermore, the editors note that a weakness in the hormonal system or stress on this system may either cause or precipitate asthma. The connection of the hormone and immune systems is little known. The fact is modern research proves that a weakness in the hormonal system increases the risk for mold/fungus infection as much as 1000-fold. This is largely because the hormonal system controls metabolic rate. Any weakening in the hormonal system leads to a reduction in the metabolic rate. The lowered metabolic rate causes a drop in body temperature, which favors the growth of molds and fungi.

An old book, written in the 1930s, gives clear evidence of how atrocious the modern medical treatment is. The author notes that as a general rule physicians in the early part of the

20th century regarded asthma as "never fatal." The number of deaths in a year amounted to less than perhaps a few dozen. Compare this to the thousands who die yearly in the United States alone. Thus, the current medical treatment regimen for asthma is an utter failure. In fact, it is a debacle.

Treatment protocol

Oregacyn is invaluable for asthma. Its active ingredients are both antihistaminic as well as antiseptic. Plus, these ingredients offer the ability to halt the production of excess mucous, while helping dislodge mucous plugs. Both Oregacyn and oil of wild Oreganol are mold killers. According to research conducted by the federal government molds are rapidly destroyed by spice extracts. Extracts of Oregano were found to be the most potent of all. Take Oregacyn, 2 capsules twice daily. Oil of wild Oreganol is also highly effective. Take three or more drops under the tongue as needed. During an acute attack take it more frequently, even every few minutes. Fortunately, it is a spice and, thus, may be taken aggressively for short term use. In reasonable amounts, like a few capsules daily, it can be taken over a prolonged period or even indefinitely. However, even though it is only made from natural wild spices, it is still potent. Thus, when taking large amounts or if taking it routinely, it is a good idea to take a natural, healthy bacteria supplement. In such circumstances take the healthy bacteria supplement, Health-Bac, right before bedtime. Health-Bac contains the most well researched type of healthy bacteria known. This European source product is backed by decades of research. It is exceptionally safe and well tolerated. Research indicates that implantation of these bacteria is superior during sleep. Thus, take probiotic supplements, i.e. natural bacteria, right before bedtime.

Raw honey may also be taken during an asthma attack. It provides energy and nutrients in an absorbable form, so direly needed to reverse this crisis. There is a contraindication: severe fungal infection, that is if the body is colonized by yeasts and fungi, which feed off of various sugars. The sugars in honey could cause a minor aggravation, although in the case of the wild oregano honey this is unusual. However, in such a case try adding a few drops of the Oreganol in the honey. This will help neutralize any sugar sensitivity.

Yet, in most instances high grade raw honeys greatly aid the asthmatic through their ability to cleanse the lungs. Such honeys exhibit soothing properties upon the respiratory tract. Crude raw honey is an excellent aid to releasing mucous. Plus, it is a natural immune tonic, in fact, it directly kills germs. It also helps sooth sore throat, while preventing or halting cough. The regular intake of such honeys can prevent mucous plugs. With wild honeys the bees are never fed sugar. Thus, these types of honeys are significantly more potent than the commercial types. Such honeys are also unheated, and, thus, they retain their full complement of enzymes. The enzymes in raw honey are the most critical agents. If by heating or processing they are rendered useless, then it is no longer medicinal. For a 100% wild medicinal honey call 1-800-243-5242 or in Canada 905-634-9428.

Asthmatics usually suffer from impaired hormonal function. In particular, their adrenal glands are often weak. Thus, in order to eradicate this condition it is crucial to restore the health of these glands. The adrenal glands are weakened by stress. They are also weakened by poor diet. If an imbalance of a significant degree develops within these glands, they frequently become infected by parasites, bacteria, and, particularly, fungi. In addition, tuberculosis readily develops in these glands, although this is almost impossible to diagnose. This makes sense, since asthma, being a lung disease, may be associated with a chronic low-grade TB infection. What's more, many authorities regard TB as a type of bacteria-fungus, and it is well known that fungi are the primary cause of asthma. Yet, low-grade TB is generally non-contagious. However, it is serious enough to cause disability and/or death. Thus, individuals with weak adrenal glands, as represented by chronic exhaustion, weakness, depression, anxiety, chronic pain, and similar debilitating symptoms, may have as an origin of their sickness chronic adrenal gland tuberculosis. One notable symptom is persistent mid-back pain in the kidney region. Another is a high vulnerability to serious infections, which, when they occur, are difficult to defeat.

Oregacyn is the ideal tonic for reversing this. Take it regularly for several months or until the symptoms are eliminated. The tremendous powers of Oregacyn are illustrated by the following case history:

> Ms. M., a 30 year old white female, had been plagued with asthma since childhood. Mothered to death by both her mother and doctors, she was over-medicated, leading to a condition known as Cushing's Syndrome. This syndrome was due to the over-use of cortisone and Prednisone and left her blown up with water and weight. Normally a size two, she is now a size twenty. Ms. M. had constant wheezing. A friend recommended Oregacyn. Only one capsule twice daily gave her enormous relief. A colleague at work told her that after taking the Oregacyn it was the first time she noticed that she

wasn't wheezing. Within five days the improvement was so dramatic that she was able to aggressively exercise at the gym without wheezing. Her mother noticed how well she was doing and broke down, crying. By consuming less than a bottle of Oregacyn, Ms. M. can safely say that her drug-resistant asthma is essentially cured.

Berylliosis

Beryllium is a metal which is usually regarded as non-toxic. However, when dust from this metal is inhaled, it causes extensive lung damage. The damage is represented by scarring, which disables the ability of the lungs to supply oxygen.

The most prominent early symptom of berylliosis is severe shortness of breath, usually occurring only with exertion. This gradually worsens until, eventually, the shortness of breath is continuous. As the disease progresses the lungs fail to supply sufficient oxygen: the individual becomes cyanotic, which means the red blood cells are unable to deliver sufficient oxygen to the tissues. Thus, the lips and fingernails become discolored (bluish). What's more the heart is adversely affected, and it gradually weakens as the disease progresses. As a result of the weakened heart and lungs fatigue and exhaustion become extreme. Ultimately, the progressive weakness and shortness of breath become debilitating. Normal activities become impossible. Memory loss may develop due to a lack of oxygen.

Treatment protocol

Edible essential spice oils are natural anti-inflammatory agents, plus they possess significant solvent properties. This solvent action aids in the mobilization of the beryllium particles so they may be extracted from the lungs. Oil of wild oregano is particularly valuable, since it is a known lymph-mobilizing agent. Take five or more drops of Oreganol three times daily. In a severe crisis take five or more drops every hour. Also, take the respiratory formula of spice extracts, that is Oregacyn, two or more capsules twice daily. The Oregacyn is critical for this condition. For tough cases take larger amounts, like three capsules three times daily (with meals).

Scar tissue may be mobilized, that is dissolved. This may be accomplished through potent fruit enzymes. Papayas and pineapples produce respectively papain and bromelain, which are aggressive protein-dissolving and anti-inflammatory enzymes. Scar tissue is protein, mainly collagen. Research proves that high potency papain and bromelain dissolve such tissue, even in the living body. Don't make the assumption that scar tissue is permanent. When given the appropriate tools, the body can mobilize scar tissue. Bromazyme is a combination of high grade papain and bromelain, the highest dosage and potency available. Experience has proven that this enzyme combination is more effective than the commercial type. Bromazyme is a pharmaceutical-grade potency, yet it is completely natural.

Blastomycoses

This is a fungal infection that occurs mainly in regions with a moist climate. It is a serious disease and often causes fatalities. The infection attacks the lungs as well as skin. From the lungs it may enter the bloodstream, causing systemic infection. It occurs mainly in states with large river valleys, like Ohio, Iowa, Missouri, Mississippi, Kentucky, Minnesota, and Illinois. It is also found in the northern part of the Midwest as well as eastern Canada.

Treatment protocol

Oregacyn multiple spice extract is the ideal treatment for this condition. Take two or more capsules twice daily. Also, take oil of wild oregano, five to ten drops twice daily. This is a serious fungal disease, and, thus, it may be necessary to take Super Strength oil of Oreganol. For difficult cases take 20 or more drops of the Super Strength twice daily.

Consume high amounts of natural vitamin C in the form of fresh orange/grapefruit juice or unsweetened currant juice (i.e. Currant-C). Made from organic mountain grown black currants, it is the ideal vitamin C-rich juice and is an excellent alternative to citrus juices. Eat plenty of vitamin C-rich foods such as oranges, grapefruit, kiwi fruit, broccoli, and strawberries. The reason for consuming natural instead of synthetic is that the natural is utilized and retained in the tissues to a greater degree. What's more, it is free of side effects. Crude natural vitamin C supplements are helpful. The only one that contains absolutely no synthetic vitamin C is Flavin-C. Flavin-C is a unique supplement. As a natural vitamin C source take two or three capsules twice daily. Selenium helps the immune system cleanse fungus: take 300 mcg of organic selenium twice daily.

Blood clots

Blood clots may originate in the lungs, or they may arise from within the veins. They may travel from exterior regions and lodge in the lungs, causing potentially fatal reactions. Thus, blood clots are one of the most serious of all conditions.

This condition is thought to arise from excessive thickness or stickiness of the blood. However, trauma, which may cause internal bleeding and clotting, is an exceptionally common cause. An even more insidious cause is jet airliner flying. This is because flying at high altitudes causes a sort of compression of the tissues, leading to sludging. It also causes dehydration, which aggravates the dilemma. There have been a rash of cases of severe and even fatal blood clots resulting from flying. By far, this most commonly occurs from flying for prolonged periods, and mostly in those flying coach, that is in cramped quarters, where there is little tendency to move about, with the middle or window seat being the most confining. People are often embarrassed or shy to impose upon others. However, for individuals taking prolonged flights movement is crucial in order to prevent stagnation of blood and, therefore, blood clotting. Thus, it is mandatory on any prolonged flight to get out of the seat and move about in the aisle. Walk in the aisles as much as possible. Move the legs and arms up and down. While seated, move the ankles and feet in an up and down pumping motion. As another preventive exercise curl up the toes. These efforts alone may prevent clot formation. Plus, avoid all alcoholic as well as caffeinated beverages. Sugar and chocolate must also be strictly avoided. Sugar, chocolate, and alcohol have a tendency to cause sludging of the blood. Alcohol is particularly harmful. It is well known that alcohol causes strokes. Therefore, on long-haul flights this substance should be strictly avoided. Why take the risk when in such a compromised circumstance?

The medical treatment for clots is potent blood thinners, which may prove lifesaving. Yet, there are a wide range of natural substances with blood thinning properties. What's more, the latter are free of serious side effects. Some of these natural compounds are even capable of dissolving clots, including the deep clots found in the deepest recesses of the lungs or legs, as is seen by the following case history:

> Mr. S., a Native American of large build, developed a severely swollen calf after a thigh/pelvic injury. Incredibly, doctors diagnosed his lower leg pain as a ruptured achilles tendon. Therefore, they caste the leg, which was a dangerous thing to do. This led to further swelling. He was then correctly guided to take a high grade fruit enzyme product, pharmaceutical-grade Bromazyme, and the dosage was 4 capsules twice daily on an empty stomach. He also took the crude red grape powder (i.e. the Resvitanol), 4 capsules twice daily. Dramatically, the chronic swelling, as well as the varicose and spider veins, rapidly improved. He also noticed a 70% reduction of the problem in less than a week. He is continuing the suggested protocol and is improving daily.

Treatment protocol

Take Bromazyme, the biological plant enzyme complex, 3 to 4 capsules twice daily on an empty stomach. For huge clots increase the dose, 4 caps three times daily on an empty stomach. Also, take Resvitanol capsules, 3 or more capsules twice daily. Fish oils and vitamin E are anti-clotting. With fish oils, take 6 or more capsules daily and 400 I.U. of vitamin E daily. Or, for a totally natural source of the complete complement of vitamin E molecules take Pumpkinol (crude cold pressed pumpkinseed oil), 2 or more tablespoons daily. Or, as a source of fatty acids in capsule form take Berry Essentials, 3 capsules twice daily. Berry Essentials are unique, since the essential fatty acids are pressed from berry seeds, in this instance red and black raspberries. This fatty acid supplement is entirely cold-pressed.

No solvents or chemicals are used. Eat fatty fish, such as sardines, salmon, albacore tuna, herring, bluefish, mackerel, halibut, and trout on a weekly basis. Rub Super Strength Oreganol on any involved area as needed. Natural vitamin C also helps prevent blood clots. This is because natural vitamin C is needed to keep the arteries from degenerating. Damaged arteries form clots more readily, because they lose their elasticity. The loss of elasticity leads to stagnation of blood and, therefore, clot formation occurs. Take Flavin-C, three or more capsules twice daily. Flavin-C is fortified with the top source of natural vitamin C known, the camu-camu berry. All of the vitamin C in Flavin-C is from natural sources.

Bronchitis

This term is named after a part of the lungs known as the bronchi. The bronchi are the tubes leading from the lower throat, that is the trachea, to the lung tissue. They conduct the air we breathe into the lungs, so that the oxygen can be extracted by the blood. The entire system is known as the bronchial tree, in fact, schematically, it looks like an upside down tree. As the bronchi diminish in size, they lose their rigid character and instead become muscular. These tiny tubules are known as bronchioles. Bronchitis is inflammation of the bronchi and bronchioles. The inflammation is usually attributed to infection, although exposure to toxic chemicals and/or allergic reactions may also be the cause.

Bronchitis may develop in several forms. It may be acute, meaning it suddenly develops. Usually, it is chronic, meaning it is a persistent inflammation/infection. In mild cases only the upper part of the bronchial tree is affected. However, the inflammation and/or infection may spread into the lower bronchial tree, that is the bronchioles, and this may result in serious consequences.

Often, with bronchitis breathing is significantly restricted. It is the inflammation, soreness, difficulty breathing, and cough that are particularly debilitating. The cough may be highly distressing and racking; there is often pain and a sensation of rawness behind the breastbone. Fever is rare, but the individual may become fatigued easily. The weakness can become debilitating. Physical activity, including exercise, is often greatly impaired.

The pattern of the cough is typical. At first there is little or no sputum, but the cough is painful. Eventually, it becomes productive, and frothy whitish sputum is produced. This type of sputum may warn of fungal infection. Later, the color changes, and it may become yellow or more rarely green. A truly green sputum with a foul odor may warn of bacterial infection. When this happens, the pain of the cough is reduced. These symptoms are classic for acute or chronic bronchitis. There is a difference between this presentation and that of pneumonia. Usually, similar symptoms occur with pneumonia, but fever, chills, and sweating also develop. Plus, pneumonia frequently results in utter exhaustion, leading to a bedridden state.

Treatment protocol

Multiple spice extracts have been proven by scientific studies to kill a wide range of germs. A federal government study proved that through exposure to spice oils both molds and bacteria, major causes of bronchial conditions, were killed. As a multiple spice extract take Oregacyn, 2 or more capsules twice daily, and increase the dosage if necessary. Take also oil of wild oregano, five drops twice daily. Crude raw honey may be helpful to ease symptoms. Such honeys help liberate lung secretions, easing congestion. Plus, they are effective germicides. A rich tasting wild oregano honey is available and can only be ordered via the mail. To order call 1-800-243-5242.

Bronchiectasis

This is a disease of the bronchial tubes. It is signified by the enlargement or weakening of certain bronchial tubes, which balloon out, forming cavities. These cavities may be seen on x-ray. This is a problem, because the bronchial tubes are normally elastic, that is tight-walled. In fact, their circumscribed size enables them to maintain proper function. This allows them to remain relatively free of debris, that is the cilia along with the muscular contractions propel debris out of the lungs. However, when they balloon out, debris, secretions, and, thus, germs accumulate. Pockets develop, and the accumulated material festers, causing bad breath. Foul-smelling sputum may be produced. This may explain the cause of many cases of undiagnosed bad breath, that is chronic lung infection, usually by bacteria or fungi. Thus, if the infection is eradicated, the malodorous condition is cured.

In the 1940s it was discovered that sinus infections may induce bronchiectasis. The germs from the infected sinuses seed the bronchial tubes, causing widespread damage. The germs apparently destroy the muscular tissues of the bronchial tubes, leading to bronchiectasis. The primary responsible germs are now known: fungi. This makes sense, because fungi are notorious for their ability to produce proteolytic enzymes, which invade and destroy tissue. They are capable of digesting living proteins, including the smooth muscle which lines the bronchioles. Once this muscle is lost, there is no means for the bronchial tubes to retain their strength or shape and, therefore, they degenerate.

The original site of these fungal infections may be the teeth, from which the organisms seep into the sinuses. Invasive dentistry may rapidly spread them, leading to acute or chronic lung or sinus infections. Septic or root canal-treated teeth may also be the foci of infection. These sites of infections can seed germs directly into the lungs, causing tissue destruction. If the sinus or tooth infection remains chronic and untreated, bronchiectasis may eventually develop. The fact is invasive dentistry is a major precipitating cause of this disease. Thus, for the physician in evaluating a case of bronchiectasis it is crucial to investigate the patients' dental history.

Treatment protocol

Oregacyn is the ideal oral therapy for this condition: take one or more capsules twice daily. Also, take oil of wild oregano, three to five or more drops under the tongue twice daily. For more difficult conditions take five to ten drops twice daily. Also, take a natural-source vitamin C supplement, such as Flavin-C, six or more capsules daily. Vitamin C is needed to maintain the strength of the bronchial tubes. Vitamin A is needed for healthy bronchioles. If you have chronic lung disease and/or bronchiectasis, take 5,000 to 10,000 I.U. daily. Or, instead of the supplement, eat organic liver, six to eight ounces twice weekly. Also, to prevent oxidative damage take a crude unprocessed antioxidant extract, such as Oreganol Antioxidant Blend, ten drops under the tongue twice daily or one capsule twice daily. This will prevent toxic damage to the lung tissues due to the release of poisonous forms of oxygen or from the toxicity of synthetic chemicals. Oxidative damage is a major cause of lung tissue damage. If this damage is halted, the lungs readily heal. For septic or diseased teeth regularly apply oil of wild oregano, a few drops, rubbed high upon the gumline twice daily.

Cancer of the lungs

This is one of the greatest and most severe of all modern epidemics. Particularly common in smokers, it is also common in those exposed to secondhand smoke as well as industrial workers who are exposed to noxious fumes. Unfortunately, individuals who have never smoked are also dying from lung cancer, that is those regularly exposed to secondhand smoke.

There are two major types of lung cancer: the type that originates directly within the lungs and the metastatic type, that is the type that is seeded to them. Regarding the latter the cancer starts in the outside organs, such as the prostate, breast, intestines, or bone, and is carried to the lungs via the blood or lymph.

Lung metastases develop in millions of Americans yearly. However, these cancers may not provoke symptoms and, thus, are occasionally discovered only through routine chest X-rays.

Primary cancers usually develop within the bronchial tubes. From here they invade the lymphatics, which disseminate the cancer throughout the lungs. The lymph glands near the tumor become infiltrated by these cells. This greatly impairs lung function. Shortness of breath may develop, which is caused by the swelling of the lymph glands and from the mechanical blockage of the tumor in the bronchial tubes. Unless such a tumor is aggressively treated, it may eat through the bronchial tubes and consume the lung tissue, making it virtually impossible to breathe.

Cancer of the lungs is usually regarded as fatal. It is believed that nothing can be done about it. Yet, physicians are unaware of the immense power of natural cures. Nature offers a wide range of cancer answers. Thus, there is no need to lose hope. In fact, cancer is merely a disease, no more threatening than any other. If the proper treatment is applied, a cure can be achieved and in many instances rather rapidly. Native Americans cured thousands of cases of cancer long before modern medicine. Cancer was also cured in ancient Greece, 16th century Europe, and the Islamic Empire. The primary mode of treatment was potent medicinal herbs. Their therapies included incantations, positive thinking, the inhalation of aromatic compounds, and medicinal herbs.

Oil of wild oregano, as well as the multiple spice extract, Oregacyn, is a potent natural tonic for the lung tissues. To greatly boost the health of the lungs and cleanse them of dangerous toxins take large amounts of these tonics. The Juice of Oregano is also an invaluable tonic. Studies in Turkey indicated that it is a powerful anti-cancer agent. The juice is perhaps the most valuable anti-cancer tonic known. It delivers a special class of compounds known as oxygenated terpenes. These substances are potent anti-cancer agents.

Treatment protocol

Stress must be minimized or preferably eliminated: it is a primary cause of cancer. If you are a worrier, halt it. A great book for this purpose is Dale Carnegie's *How to Stop Worrying and Start Living*. If you smoke, stop immediately. If those close to you smoke, they should be prohibited from doing so. If they cannot stop their habit, make them smoke outdoors at a distance from the house. Cigarette smoke-tainted clothing, walls, or furniture must either be disposed of or cleansed. To achieve a complete cure the individual must be free of virtually any degree of exposure. Cigarette smoke is exceptionally toxic and is the primary chemical cause of lung cancer. Juice of Oregano has a significant anecdotal history as a cancer remedy. It is the ideal antidote for immediately reversing the toxic effects of cigarette smoke. As of yet, however, there is no government approval for such a treatment. Even so, it may be considered an immune tonic. Drink 2 to 6 ounces twice daily. Also, drink Juice of Rosemary, 4 ounces daily. Rosemary has been shown to be one of nature's most potent anti-cancer agents. Take also the multiple spice extract, that is Oregacyn, 3 capsules twice daily with meals. Increase the intake of dark green leafy vegetables and vitamin C-rich fruit, particularly organic kiwi, papaya, grapefruit, blueberries, and strawberries. Eat a large organic spinach salad daily topped with extra virgin olive oil and vinegar. Objects contaminated by cigarette smoke must be decontaminated. Use a vinegar-oregano oil cleaning solution to wash walls or other hard surfaces. To decontaminate clothes add vinegar and oregano oil to the wash cycle. Spray any smoke-contaminated rooms with Germ-a-Clenz. This may also be sprayed on clothes.

Take precautions to protect yourself against secondhand smoke. Do not consume nitrated or smoked meats: they are primary cancer promoters. Eliminate the intake of all refined vegetable oils and hydrogenated oils. Butter, tallow, and extra virgin olive oil are allowed. Furthermore, regarding spice extracts take as much as is needed to eradicate the disorder. In some cases megadoses are indicated. Regarding Juice of Oregano large amounts may be taken, such as 4 ounces twice daily. Also, take large amounts of Oreganol (Maximum Strength), 10 or more drops several times daily. The rosemary juice may also be taken in large amounts, 2 to 4 ounces twice daily. Oregano oil may also be taken profusely, like a few drops every hour.

Candida

Candida is a yeast, which infects human tissues. It is a monumental cause of human disease, disability, and even death. Candida is one of the most common pathogens of the lungs. It may infect virtually any organ, including the blood, spleen, intestines, esophagus, stomach, bladder, kidneys, and even the brain.

Candida has been implicated in a number of respiratory diseases, particularly asthma, sinusitis, ear infections, and bronchitis. It may also cause a type of pneumonia, which is usually fatal. This is particularly true of post-surgical and hospitalized patients, who may readily suffer from a potentially fatal form of Candidal pneumonia.

While it is difficult to kill via the standard medical therapy, research proves that spice extracts are highly effective against it. Preliminary research indicates that such extracts are just as effective as the standard drugs.

The components of Oregacyn kill Candida. The fact that spice oil extracts kill Candida was proven by Georgetown University. The extracts were so effective that they were shown in preliminary research to completely clear yeasts from organs and tissues, while improving the health of the test animals. Within 30 days all traces of this yeast were purged from the test animals. This indicates that the P73 wild oregano oil exhibited an antifungal effect equally as potent as pharmaceutical drugs. Yet, its value is far greater than any drug. This is because wild oregano extract is non-toxic. Thus, they can be used repeatedly without harm.

Treatment protocol

Take a multiple spice extract, that is Oregacyn, two capsules twice daily. Also, take oil of wild Oreganol, five to ten drops under the tongue twice daily. For difficult cases use the Super Strength oil of oregano, five or more drops under the tongue twice daily. For tough conditions increase the amount to a dropperful (25 drops) three times daily.

Chlorine gas inhalation

This is becoming an increasingly common illness. As a gas it is one of the most caustic substances known. This disaster can occur industrially, that is via a major toxic spill, or individually, that is through exposure to commercially available chlorine. Chlorine is one of the most potent synthetic chemicals known, both as a gas and liquid. Yet, its destructive properties are enhanced when the liquid form converts to a gas. This conversion readily occurs, usually as a consequence of toxic spills or accidental release from factories. Plus, it is used in virtually every home in North America, so toxic reactions are common.

Virtually every household has experienced some type of chlorine accident or exposure. Such an exposure usually leads to irritation, and/or burns, even organ damage or death. The lungs are particularly vulnerable to chlorine-induced toxicity. This is why it is crucial to know its natural antidotes, since there are no drugs to neutralize its toxicity.

Treatment protocol

In the event of sudden toxic exposure cover all respiratory passages with whatever is available, preferably a mask. Also, wear protective clothing. However, if unavailable, use a soft cloth. Take Oreganol Antioxidant Blend, ten or more drops under the tongue as often as every few minutes. Reduce the dosage as soon as the danger is reversed to a maintenance of ten to twenty drops (one dropperful) twice daily. Also, take Oregacyn, one or more capsules twice daily. For chlorine-induced skin damage apply oil of wild oregano once or twice daily. In the event of severe chlorine burns make a salve from wild Mediterranean honey, that is thistle or oregano honey, along with a few drops of oregano oil or preferably the antioxidant form of this oil (Oreganol Antioxidant Blend): apply to skin and cover with Telfa pad or gauze. Repeat as needed until skin is completely healed.

Colds

No one knows for sure what causes the common cold. What is known is that it is an infectious disease, probably a virus.

However, recent evidence points to the role of fungi and fungal toxins in causing cold, as well as flu, symptoms.

Theories for the cause of colds originated thousands of years ago. A book written in the early 1900s, *How to Get Well*, by Dr. W. A. Evans, offers some insight into past and, seemingly viable, theories. Here is what Emeritus Eliot in this book said in the early 1900s:

> "People who live in the forest, in open barns, or with open windows do not catch cold...(colds are)...caused by impure air, lack of exercise, or overeating." The naturalist John Muir observed, "as long as I camp out in the mountains without tents or blankets, I get along very well, but the very minute I get into a house and have a warm bed and begin to live on fine food, I get into a draft and the first thing I know I am coughing and sneezing and threatened with (infection)."

Also, at the turn of the century Irving Foster noted that people who live outdoors are virtually immune from colds. A chart is listed showing the incidence of colds/flu. Their findings were as follows: impure air causes respiratory diseases. They failed to determine the culprit, but they did discern much of the cause. Pneumonia and bronchitis were found to occur mainly in the winter, when people "house themselves up and breathe the foul air of unventilated rooms."

What is known is that the common cold is highly contagious. People who are indoors during the winter are the most vulnerable, since this wintry infection is readily spread by close contact, especially through coughing or sneezing. Incredibly, the infection can even be contracted from direct contact with inanimate objects such as doorknobs, railings, and utensils.

Cold victims suffer miserably, although it is a rather limited disease. It strikes the head and neck, and the nasal passages are severely affected.

That weather changes are involved in the creation of colds has been suspected since the time of Hippocrates. Most colds occur towards the middle of fall, for instance, in October. The incidence rises again in January and February, climaxing in March. During the spring and summer the incidence is low. From this it is easy to understand the role of the sun. When there is plenty of sunlight, the incidence of colds plummets. Thus, cold weather itself is not the cause of colds. People who are constantly outdoors during the winter rarely get them. For instance, in their native environment the Inuit (formerly known as Eskimos) have always been cold free. When they were originally visited by Western explorers, they caught colds from them. This shows that colds are transmissible, but it also proves that cold weather or dry cold air by itself fails to cause them. There must be other factors. For instance, while colds do develop when the weather turns cold, this is also when people spend a greater amount of time indoors. Here too the solar penetration is greatly diminished. It is also when people first turn on their furnaces after months of inactivity. Most furnaces are in basements, which are excellent repositories of dust and, particularly, mold. The fact is mold counts in houses may reach astronomically high levels as the result of forced air heat, especially if the filters are poorly cleaned and/or if the furnace is in a basement with high mold counts. When the molds are inhaled, they attach to the lung and bronchial tissues. There, they reproduce, secreting poisons known as mycotoxins. These mycotoxins are exceptionally poisonous, thus, they debilitate the immune system, increasing the vulnerability to infections by cold viruses and other pathogens. The fact is if the molds which colonize the nasal passages and sinuses were destroyed, colds would fail to occur. One noted British researcher, Dr. A. V. Hill, believes that cold weather instigates colds, because people are primarily indoors. They stay for longer periods in warm and stuffy rooms, failing to ventilate them. They perspire, giving off noxious gases. They sneeze and cough, liberating pathogens, which, if not ventilated, multiply indoors.

During cold weather people often rely on forced heat furnaces and, habitually, fail to open windows. This was confirmed by Dr. E. O. Jordan of the University of Chicago, who found that 90% of colds occur when there is minimal or no ventilation and when windows are never opened, like during the chilly part of the fall as well as the winter. This is particularly true in office buildings, where it is socially unacceptable to open windows on blustery, cold days. This is proof that a change in weather, that is a change in human habits based upon the weather, is a definite factor in causing colds. The fact is people who live and work in crowded surroundings are the primary victims. Colds simply fail to occur in remote or uncrowded environments.

Poor hygiene increases the risks for developing colds. The hands are constantly covered with the residues from, for instance, a sneeze or from touching the nasal region, mouth, etc. Then, the contaminated hand induces transmission through contact with other individuals through hugs, pats, handshakes, kisses, utensils, etc. or through touching inanimate objects, like railings or doorknobs. Thus, cold germs remain viable for at least a few hours and are readily transmitted to other individuals. The virus is active and lies in wait for its next victim.

Crowding is a major cause of colds, but this is only because it increases the ease for their spread. Germs are spread mainly through the air, arising from the breath of various humans or through sneezing or coughing. However, crowded places may also place people at risk, because of contaminated inanimate objects, including doorknobs and toilet seats.

Germs are invasive. Their objective is to attack and colonize. They lie in wait for a vulnerable subject. If you live or work in a crowded environment, place great importance upon proper hygiene. This will help minimize the potential for exposure. Many germs are spread only through close contact. Thus, careful attention to hygiene can largely prevent communicable diseases. Yet, even the most fastidious individual may fall victim to the germs found in a crowded environment. This is because most infectious diseases are airborne, and, thus, the infections may develop in spite of all precautions. This is why hygienic individuals may readily develop infections after riding on a subway or bus or flying in an airplane. In other words, the individual may be fastidious in his/her hygiene and still develops the infection simply because the air is foul. However, there is a simple solution: antiseptic protection.

Cold weather and/or being outdoors in the winter, that is being exposed to cold air, is not the main cause of colds. In fact, spending time outdoors is preventive. This is because fresh air cleanses the sinuses, lungs, in fact, the entire respiratory tract. In contrast, indoor air spreads colds, especially in the fall and winter. As stated previously one problem is that during cold weather furnaces are used. In causing sinus or cold/flu symptoms forced heat furnaces are one of the greatest villains. The dry heat desiccates the mucous membranes, weakening them.

Mucous membranes must remain moist to maintain the proper anti-viral defenses. This may be corrected by adding moisture to the air, enough to prevent drying of the membranes but not too much, which could encourage the growth of molds.

The lack of sunlight during fall/winter predisposes to colds. This is because solar rays are potent germicides. Even though there is sunlight during this time the power of the rays is significantly diminished, because of the increased distance of the sun from the earth. In other words, when sunlight is diminished, germs flourish, not so much outdoors but indoors. During the cold winter period the outdoor air is relatively sterile. However, the combination of the warmth from artificial heating plus a lack of sunlight allows germs to multiply indoors in vast numbers. There is another reason that a lack of sunlight increases the risks: a reduction in metabolism. Sunlight is needed to boost the metabolic rate. When this rate slows, the immune system is more sluggish, and blood flow is reduced. When blood flow is impaired, there is less oxygen delivered to the tissues. Oxygen is one of nature's most powerful antiseptics.

For modern medicine the treatment of colds has always been a conundrum. Vaccines have been attempted, but these have proven useless. These vaccines have been made using specific cold viruses. Their failure is in part due to the fact that colds are caused by a wide range of organisms, not just viruses.

Molds are a major cause of colds and cold-like symptoms. The molds are highly toxic to the immune system. They suppress immunity, making the body more vulnerable to viral attack. If the molds are killed, the cold virus is rendered impotent. The fact is the cold virus is dependent upon the molds to cause infections.

As early as the 1940s medical doctors recommended colon cleansing as a treatment for colds. The idea is that toxins in the colon depress the immune system, increasing the risks for infection. Enemas and laxatives were administered. These seem to have had a positive effect. Yet, it is reasonable to presume that occasional colon cleansing through herbal laxatives or enemas may aid in prevention. What's more a variety of natural tonics have been tried with modest success. In the 1940s and 50s prodigious amounts of lemonade and orange juice were recommended with definite results. The benefit is largely due to the content of immune boosting vitamins such as folic acid and vitamin C. If using lemonade, do not add sugar. Make your own lemonade from real lemons. Sweeten with raw honey or stevia. Sugar depresses immunity, prolonging the illness. The use of hot spices on the feet is a valuable and time-honored aid. I found this recommendation in a medical book written in the 1940s. The doctors recommended bathing the feet in mustard baths or soaks. This is because the hot phenolic compounds from spicy substances, such as mustard, are potent germicides, plus these substances stimulate metabolism, which is sluggish during colds. Even superior to this is the use of oil of wild oregano. In a foot soak add about 50 drops. Soak for an hour or two. Results will be noticed fairly quickly, like within two hours.

As mentioned previously a lack of fresh air is an enormous cause of disease, but, today, this is rarely recognized. People stay much of their lives indoors in poorly ventilated facilities. Some office buildings offer no access to outside air. This extreme lack of ventilation increases the risks for a variety of illnesses, including asthma, colds, flu, sinus problems, migraine headaches, bronchitis, pneumonia, and even tuberculosis.

In the past it was clearly known that stagnant, contaminated, and/or polluted air causes ill health. A book written in 1884, Smith's *Human Body and its Health*, describes how this occurs. In a section called *Waste Matters Given Off By the Lungs* a number of facts are provided. The lungs are described as a gas-exchanging organ, which siphons in oxygen and expels carbon dioxide and other useless gases. In fact, the lungs play a major role in aggressively expelling waste material. Water is also expelled with each exhalation and usually this water is permeated with noxious gases.

Incredibly, within 24 hours the average human expels through the lungs up to a pint of wastewater. When we breath, we intake a combination of mainly oxygen and nitrogen. When we exhale, the air has lost oxygen and gained carbon dioxide plus water vapor as well as various noxious and potentially toxic gases, like methane, urea, and pentane. What's more, according to Smith, who was a hygiene expert, expelled air is "not fit to be breathed again...(and it is so useless)...we could not live in it...moreover, it is injurious."

The accumulation of large amounts of this human effluent can be catastrophic. Smith describes a case in Calcutta: nearly 150 men were packed into a room only 18 x18 feet, that is the size of a large bedroom. Within 24 hours, some 120 men died. Even in 1884 Smith regarded fresh air as a rare commodity, stating that virtually everyone living in the modern world suffers constantly from a lack of it and that its importance should continuously be kept in mind. Vague symptoms, he says, due to a lack of fresh air, are likely such as a general sensation of illness, mental fatigue, drowsiness, and lack of desire to exercise. A few deep breaths of the fresh air outdoors could quickly regenerate the health and eliminate the symptoms.

Treatment protocol

Extracts of wild and mountain-harvested spices are potential cures for the common cold. In fact, colds are no contest for the nasal and sinus cleansing powers of Oregacyn as well as oregano oil. Indeed, the positive experiences of hundreds of thousands of individuals prove that oil of Oreganol and similar spice extracts cure the common cold. The fact is the antiviral actions of this oil are indisputable. What's more, crude spice extracts are a type of general germicide, capable of destroying cold viruses and flu viruses as well as molds. Thus, all the various causes of cold/flu syndrome are resolved.

Oregano, cinnamon, cloves, and sage are potent antihistaminic substances, plus they contain compounds, notably terpenes, long chain alcohols, flavonoids, and phenolic agents, which boost the body's anti-viral defenses. Oregacyn multiple spice extract, rich in antiseptic spices, including sage, cumin, and oregano, is a dependable means to obliterate cold symptoms. Yet, more importantly it obliterates the germs which instigate it. The fact is Oregacyn is a certain cure for the common cold. Take 1 or 2 capsules three times daily with meals. For severe cases increase the dose, for instance, 2 to 3 capsules four times daily with meals (or food). Also, oil of wild oregano is useful. For best results take the oil frequently, like every few hours. Also, rub the oil on the feet morning and night. Foot rubs with hot spices have been used successfully in the treatment of colds for hundreds of years.

Raw honey is an excellent medicine for respiratory conditions, particularly colds. According to Loran in *Health Through Rational Diet* honey's content of antibiotic acids, particularly formic acid, accounts for much of its antiseptic qualities. Plus, formic acid is apparently an antidote for excessive mucous and is very soothing for clearing the throat and sinuses. Honey is certainly a sugar, but it is the most natural type available. It is readily digested and causes less stress upon the body than refined sugar. Its source is the nectar from flowers. The flowers contain various nutritive and antibiotic substances, which the bees concentrate. The formic acid is synthesized by the bees, which secrete it into the honey.

The antiseptic and medicinal properties of honey are largely dependent upon the type of plants visited by the bees. Honeys derived from wild plants, especially plants growing in remote regions, are ideal. A wild oregano honey is available. Made from oregano and other antiseptic plants, it is exceptionally rich in organic acids, such as formic acid, as well as minerals. It is a dark colored honey, indicating the intensity of its mineral content. It is a high mountain source and is free of all chemicals. Wild oregano honey may be ordered via mail order: 1-800-243-5242.

Hot lemonade may also be a useful tonic. Do not add sugar; either drink it unsweetened straight, or sweeten it with raw honey. To make this thoroughly squeeze the juice of four lemons and add a quart of water. Also, add a pinch of sea salt. Sweeten with honey to desired sweetness, and drink a quart daily.

Avoid all solid food. Colds are aggravated by eating dense foods, like meat, cheese, butter, eggs, as well as rich sauces. Eat lightly and the cold will dissipate quickly. Helpful foods are salad greens, citrus fruit, citrus juices, and broth soups.

Collapsed lung

This serious condition is becoming increasingly common. It is usually caused by trauma. However, infection may also cause it.

The lungs are highly resistant to collapse. This is because they are a tough elastic organ. They have a natural tendency to stay inflated. This is because the lungs are surrounded by a vacuum, which keeps them inflated. However, if this vacuum is compromised, the lungs may collapse. This usually occurs from direct trauma. However, certain lung diseases, as well as sudden infections, may damage the outer lung layers, and a defect may develop, breaking the vacuum.

A type of collapsed lung may occur in tuberculosis. It happens without warning. It is caused by the ulceration of the outer layers of the lung, which destroys the natural vacuum. This usually occurs in people over 45.

Another type develops in younger people, including athletes. It also occurs without warning. Healthy college students are the usual victims. It begins with a sudden episode of chest pain, difficulty breathing, and, eventually, cyanosis. A smoldering unknown lung infection may have precipitated it, although excessive alcohol intake and/or binge drinking may be the primary precipitant. Alcohol damages the lungs' protective coating, causing these organs to be more vulnerable to collapse. Plus, alcohol destroys vitamins C and E, needed to maintain the lungs' structural integrity.

Treatment protocol

Vitamin C may prevent the breakdown of the outer lung layers. It is also needed to maintain the integrity of its elastic components. A lack of vitamin C leads to the breakdown of lung tissues. Take a crude natural vitamin C, such as Flavin-C, three capsules twice daily. Oreganol Antioxidant Blend is an invaluable lung tonic. Rich in potent antioxidants it helps rapidly regenerate damaged lung tissues. Take 10 or more drops twice daily. To cleanse the lungs of infection take oil of wild oregano, 10 or more drops twice daily. Fatty acids, such as lecithin and essential fatty acids, may help re-inflate the lungs by providing those slippery substances known as surfactants. Take lecithin, 3 heaping tablespoons daily. As a source of crude essential fatty acids as well as vitamin E take Pumpkinol (crude mountainous pumpkinseed oil), three tablespoons daily. Or, if capsules are preferred take Berry Essentials, 2 or 3 caps twice daily. Also, take fish oils, 6 to 10 capsules daily. Oregacyn may also prove helpful: take 1 or 2 capsules twice daily.

Congestive heart failure

This condition is manifested essentially by water-logging of the body. It is due usually to a weakened heart, which fails to efficiently pump blood. The blood backs up and, thus, fluids accumulate in the body, including in the lungs. However, it may start as lung disease. In other words, the lungs could be damaged, and this places extensive pressure on the heart, weakening it and leading to the accumulation of fluids and secretions in the lungs. The latter is particularly common in a condition known as pulmonary fibrosis, that is scarring of the lungs. Regardless of the cause in this condition the lungs are flooded with secretions and fluids, which can rapidly result in fatality.

The key to reversing this is to improve the function of the heart as well as the lungs. Thus, the following protocol aids in strengthening both of these critical organs.

Treatment protocol

To strengthen the heart take crude red grape flavonoids, (i.e. Resvitanol) a heaping teaspoon three times daily. To strengthen the lungs take Oregacyn, 2 capsules two or three times daily with meals. Raw honey can be an immense aid. Consume wild oregano honey, which is rich in heart-nourishing trace minerals, a quarter cup or more daily. The honey greatly improves the osmotic pressure in the blood, preventing fluid back up. Add sea salt to the diet, at least a teaspoon daily. Take a natural thyroid-supporting supplement, such as ThyroKelp, three or more capsules twice daily. The thyroid gland is crucial for maintaining a strong heart. Also, take crude royal jelly capsule (i.e. Royal Kick), four capsules every morning. Oil of oregano strengthens both the lungs and heart: take 3 to 5 drops under the tongue twice daily. Yet, the Oregano Juice is perhaps the most critical therapy. Researchers in the Middle East determined that it greatly improves the pumping power of the heart. To reverse congestive heart failure take Juice of Oregano, two ounces twice daily.

Cough

A cough is merely a symptom. It may be generated by a vast number of illnesses or conditions. Cough can be an extremely serious symptom, signaling potentially fatal disease of the lungs. Or, it may be caused by something completely innocuous such as excessive wax build-up in the ears.

Usually, suppressing a cough, that is halting it with potent sedative medications, is a bad idea. The cough may be a good sign, that is that the body is attempting to rid itself of toxins, germs, or irritants. If the noxious agent is eradicated, the cough disappears. Thus, the cause of the cough should be resolved and/or the irritant should be cleansed. Though wild oregano may eliminate a cough, it does so by eradicating the most common cause: germs.

Treatment protocol

Chronic cough is a signal that something is irritating the lungs, usually allergens, toxic chemicals, or microbes. Oregacyn is a natural antioxidant, anti-allergen, anti-toxin, and anti-microbial. It possesses potent anti-cough powers, a property known as antitussive. Oregacyn is perhaps the most potent antitussive agent known.

> **Case History:** While I was giving a lecture a woman in the front row was coughing uncontrollably. In fact, she kept interrupting the lecture. I passed her a bottle of Oreganol and told her to take a few drops under the tongue. Within seconds the cough stopped. Later, she noted that, amazingly, she'd had the cough for ten years and no other medicine had helped her. She left the lecture with teary eyes, utterly grateful for the power of wild oregano.

To eradicate the cause of the cough take 2 capsules twice daily. For severe unrelenting cough take higher amounts, like 2 or 3 capsules three times daily.

Raw honey, especially antiseptic honeys, like wild thistle and oregano honeys, may be helpful. Certainly, the raw honey will help soothe the throat and is ideal for throat irritation due to repeated coughing. The honey may be taken directly, like a teaspoon melted into the mouth or in warm herbal tea. Or, it may be stirred into warm salt water or vinegar water and used as a gargle.

Cystic fibrosis

This is a hereditary disease of certain glands in the body known as exocrine glands, that is the glands that secrete digestive juices, mucus, tears, etc. The main gland affected is the pancreas, however, the function of the lungs is also severely compromised. This is because in cystic fibrosis there is a defect in mucus secretion. The mucus is extremely sticky and thick, which causes a wide range of disabilities. This thick mucus plugs the various ducts, leading to swelling, scarring, and permanent damage. The organs become so damaged that they fail to produce their secretions. For instance, the pancreas fails to produce enzymes, and the lungs fail to produce sufficient quantities of protective mucus. The thick mucus which is produced is abnormal in chemistry. It fails to protect the lungs from germs, plus it plugs various lung tubules, allowing germs to multiply. The lack of enzymes impairs digestion, leading to malnutrition and outright vitamin deficiency.

The digestion of fat is particularly impaired, which leads to a deficiency of fat soluble vitamins, notably vitamins A, E, and D. The lack of vitamin A is of particular concern, since this vitamin is required for the creation of healthy lung cells and for protecting the lungs against infection.

In cystic fibrosis virtually all of the organs are negatively affected. The greatest disruption occurs in the exocrine glands. "Exo" means exterior. Thus, the exocrine glands are the ones which secrete their productions outward. For instance, the pancreas produces enzymes, which it secretes into the intestines. Its function is greatly impaired in cystic fibrosis. Other glands which produce outgoing secretions include the sweat glands, mucous glands, breasts, and salivary glands. All of these glands fail to produce sufficient quantities of excretions, plus they tend to degenerate, becoming scarred or plugged. This plugging, which occurs in the ducts of these various glands, is the key feature of this disease. Clogged ducts breed germs. Thus, infections are the major cause of illness and death. This demonstrates that the key to aiding these individuals is to keep the secretions flowing and prevent scar formation.

The sweat glands are also negatively affected. These glands lose their ability to reabsorb salt. Thus, salt is readily lost, and salt deficiency, that is a deficiency of sodium and chloride, is common. The lack of sodium and chloride greatly disturbs body function. Thus, the regular intake of large amounts of salt helps prevent a variety of complications.The fact is salt, as sea salt, must be a regular additive to the diet.

For individuals to remain as healthy as possible aggressive care is necessary. In the past the death rate was exceedingly high, with victims usually dying by early adulthood. However, today with proper care sufferers can live a relatively normal life. Nutritional and herbal remedies have had an enormously positive impact upon the course of this disease. Without proper supplementation and dietary measures cystic fibrosis patients rapidly degenerate. Mechanical aids, such as breathing exercises, massage, and respiratory therapies, are also useful, since they assist greatly in keeping the secretions flowing and preventing mucous plugs. It may also be helpful to naturally bolster thyroid function. This is because this gland controls both excretory actions as well as the quality and consistency of body secretions.

Treatment protocol

Oil of wild Oreganol is critical for this condition and may often prove lifesaving. Oregacyn is also particularly valuable, as it helps cleanse the body of deep-seated pathogens. Use also the oil as a foot massage; there are hundreds of lung reflexes there. Rub preferably the Super Strength oil of Oreganol on the feet once or twice daily. After rubbing it on the feet in the morning, put on stockings. This will hold the oil on the region, offering a sort of daylong therapy.

Vitamin-mineral therapy is essential, as is the intake of fatty acids. Fat soluble vitamins and fatty acids must be taken in a mycelized form. Also, a mycelized form of wild oregano oil is now available. This water-soluble form is ideal for cystic fibrosis victims, since it is easily absorbed. For more information call 1-800-243-5242.

Salt depletion is common and dangerous. Sea salt should be routinely added to food. A high quality kelp supplement, such as ThyroKelp, should be taken on a daily basis (2 to 10 capsules daily). For infants or small children such capsules may be opened and added to food. Kelp is a rich source of iodine, sodium, and chloride, which are direly needed by cystic fibrosis patients. Commercial kelp is often contaminated with high levels of arsenic. The kelp in ThyroKelp has been assayed and shown to be free of significant levels of such industrial contaminants.

A high protein diet has been found to be the most beneficial for this condition. Refined carbohydrates, such as white flour, rice, and sugar, must be strictly avoided. The fact is grains are the most difficult of all foods to digest and, thus, should be restricted or avoided completely. Corn and beans should also be avoided. This is because such foods commonly cause allergic intolerance, plus they are high in substances called lectins. The lectins cause irritation of the mucous membranes. The ideal diet is rich in fresh fish, red meat, poultry, fresh vegetables, and fresh fruit. Milk products that may be tolerated include yogurt and goat's milk. Eggs may also be tolerated. Buy only free-range or organic eggs. Although milk and eggs are nutritionally rich, allergic reactions to these foods are common and, thus, they may need to be avoided. If milk is strictly restricted, be sure to provide a calcium supplement as well as supplemental vitamin D. However, opt for pure organic whole milk. This is usually tolerated, even by cystic fibrosis sufferers. If cow's milk is poorly tolerated, use whole goat's milk.

The diet should be free of foods which clog intestinal function, that is foods which are difficult to digest. Grains are among the most difficult of all foods to digest. As mentioned previously this is partly because grains contain lectins, which are sticky substances that become glue-like within the intestines. Lectins utterly disrupt the digestive tracts of celiac and/or cystic fibrosis victims. They should be thoroughly avoided. In this respect high-protein foods, such as meats, eggs, and whole milk, are far superior, since they are devoid of lectins.

Many individuals have extreme difficulty digesting grains. Celiac disease is a specific syndrome in which the ingestion of grains destroys the intestinal lining. In this syndrome individuals develop toxic reactions to any grains which contain the protein known as gluten. This is one of the few diseases that is much like cystic fibrosis in its presentation. Ideally, for cystic fibrosis patients all gluten-containing grains, that is wheat, oats, rye, kamut, spelt, and barley, should be strictly avoided. Interestingly, the aforementioned grains are also high in lectins. Corn and beans, which are also high in lectins (but contain no gluten), should also be avoided. It is crucial in this disease to strictly avoid grains. Perhaps cystic fibrosis is a type of toxicity due to grain intolerance.

Demolition lung (World Trade Center Syndrome)

It has been long known that workers in the demolition field suffer a specific respiratory syndrome. This is due to the inhalation of the dust liberated from construction and demolition.

A similar syndrome has resulted from the World Trade Center disaster. This debacle resulted in the liberation of vast quantities of airborne particles, many of them poisonous. Asbestos, silica, lead, cadmium, volatile hydrocarbons, petrochemical fumes: all were liberated. Obviously, the people in the inner city inhaled these substances in relatively large quantities. The plumes of dust and fumes floated throughout the city, contaminating the lungs of hundreds of thousands of people. The result may be thousands of cases of chronic lung disease: a dangerous and insidious epidemic.

According to the *Chicago Tribune* workers, as well as residents, near the disaster site have become increasingly ill. The dust and toxins released by the collapsing towers have made them ill, creating fears of long-term diseases such as emphysema, asthma, and lung cancer. In fact, these fears are real. Anyone who worked on the site and failed to use a respirator is at a high risk for inhalation-related illnesses, including asbestosis, silicosis, heavy metal toxicity, and lung infection.

Asbestos is especially dangerous. However, the dust of vaporized concrete is particularly vile. Imagine what this must do to to the lungs. Finely milled concrete flour in the air is inhaled into the moist lungs. The concrete dust, rich in silica and other damaging minerals, mixed with the moisture within the lungs congeals into a concrete-like compound, causing massive lung irritation and leading to swelling, inflammation, and scarring.

The Trade Center site is asbestos-contaminated. In fact, contamination by asbestos in lower Manhattan is rife. The authorities cannot be relied on in their lackadaisical attitude. It is obviously contaminated. The 1970s era building made extensive use of asbestos in pipe insulation and for other purposes. The vaporization of any such massive site must lead to serious pollution, since today's high-rise buildings contain billions of pounds of hazardous materials. Government firms may have seemingly minimal concern for the level of contamination. In contrast, reputable private firms have discovered that the levels are exceptionally high, as would be expected from the types and age of the involved buildings. Informing the public of the level of poison is helpful, not harmful.

Certain agencies have reported that air in lower Manhattan is safe. Yet, thousands of New York City residents are reporting lung symptoms, all of which have developed since the collapse. Even so, the authorities continue to minimize its scope, supposedly to avoid creating panic. In fact, it is less stressful to admit the existence of a problem, even if there is little the government can do about it. For instance, local doctors in inner Manhattan are convinced that the air is poisonous. Dr. Stephen Levin, medical director of occupational and environment diseases at Mount Sinai Medical Center, claims that the air is causing serious respiratory ailments. The fact is nearly half of all rescue workers, some 5,000 individuals, developed chronic lung symptoms as a result of persistently inhaling the toxic and dust-contaminated air. This degree of contamination is causing a significant syndrome, which will likely plague thousands of individuals for years, perhaps lifetimes. This illustrates the importance of utilizing natural healing aids to assist the ability of the lungs to heal. What's more, according to the WB11 News thousands of New York City firemen and women are suffering from a constellation of respiratory symptoms, which, because of their timing and unusual nature, have been coined The World Trade Center Syndrome.

As a result of exposure to these toxins long term damage is likely, and a thorough understanding of the causes of this syndrome could help prevent disability as well as premature death. As a result, ultimately, much agony, as well as many lives, will be saved.

The appropriate action must be taken to reverse the forthcoming health crises. In fact, without effective or curative treatment, potentially hundreds of thousands of New York City residents could develop chronic debilitating lung diseases.

Even with the degree of poisoning experienced by New York City residents permanent pain and agony is unnecessary. This is because certain natural compounds speed the healing of lung tissue and also protect it from further damage. Such compounds can also aid in the removal of noxious compounds.

Treatment protocol

Massive doses of certain natural herbs, spices, vitamins, minerals, and antioxidants are required to reverse the damage. The following protocol is specific for the degree of damage suffered by the residents as a result of the trade center collapse: Beta carotene (natural source only): 50,000 to 75,000 I.U. daily. Take this dosage for two months, then reduce the amount to 25,000 I.U. daily. Be sure you take a 100% natural source of beta carotene.

Organic selenium: 400 to 600 mcg daily. Note: this must be the organic or amino acid-bound type. Do not use sodium selenite or selenious acid. These synthetic types are potentially toxic.

Vitamin E: 800 I.U. daily (or, for a more powerful antioxidant action, take edible oil of wild rosemary, 10 drops twice daily).

Vitamin C: 1000 mg daily. Note: for optimal benefits take a natural type of vitamin C supplement. Crude natural vitamin C offers infinitely greater healing powers than the synthetic. Take Flavin-C, four capsules twice daily.

Oreganol P73 oil of wild oregano: take five to ten drops under the tongue twice daily. Take more if needed, like five to 10 drops four times daily. For difficult situations use the Super Strength oil of wild oregano at the same dosages.

Oregacyn spice blend is also extremely valuable, ideal for reversing severe respiratory syndromes. Take one or two capsules twice daily. In the case of individuals working directly in the demolition or disaster environment and/or who have developed persistent lung symptoms, take larger amounts, like 2 or 3 capsules twice daily. Usually, benefits are noted within days.

Vitamin C-rich foods are lung-friendly. Eat kiwi fruit, oranges, grapefruit, lemons, and limes as often as possible. In particular, eat fresh organic oranges, two daily. If unavailable drink organic fresh-frozen orange juice, one or more pints daily. Hot, spicy foods are also lung-friendly. Use cayenne, curry powder, horseradish, oregano, rosemary, cilantro, coriander, and similar spicy/hot substances. A recent USDA study (2002) proves that spices are by far the most powerful antioxidants. Incredibly, of all spices oregano was the most powerful. According to the USDA it "blew away" the competition. The oregano proved to be 40 times more powerful than apples and some 5 times more powerful than antioxidant-rich blueberries. Chicken soup made with large amounts of garlic and onion, as well as a teaspoon or two of wild oregano, helps clear and heal the lungs. Add to the diet plenty of nutrient-rich vegetables such as broccoli, Brussel's sprouts, cauliflower, spinach, red sweet peppers, and green peppers. Strictly avoid cigarette smoke. If you are a smoker, quit.

Emphysema

This is one of the most devastating of all lung diseases. It is manifested by total destruction of lung cells, that is the alveoli.

The lung is an elastic organ. Under a microscope tiny air organs are revealed, which expand and contract with every breath. These are known as the air vesicles or alveoli. It is a beautiful sight to watch these microscopic organs expand and contract with every inhalation and exhalation.

The alveoli are highly vulnerable to toxic insults. In particular cigarette smoke readily destroys them. There are tens of billions of alveoli, yet, if enough of the alveoli are destroyed, emphysema develops. Thus, emphysema is defined as the loss of the normal elastic cells of the lungs. When these cells are destroyed, the lung enlarges, pushing the ribs out. That is why emphysema patients are barrel chested.

It is a little known fact that germs can cause or accelerate emphysema. Mold is one of the most insidious toxins that can cause it. Certain molds are highly invasive, that is they aggressively attack and destroy tissue. Plus, molds produce mycotoxins, which aggressively destroy lung cells. The molds themselves destroy human cells. They may, in fact, feed off of them, including the nutrient-rich lung cells. What's more, molds secrete enzymes, which digest, that is destroy, human tissue. Thus, they must be aggressively destroyed for a cure to be achieved.

With emphysema victims there is yet another dilemma: oxidative damage to the lungs. This may be evidence that the body and specifically the lung tissue is deficient in critical antioxidants such as selenium, glutathione, vitamin C, and vitamin E. Antioxidants limit and, in some instances, reverse the oxidative damage occurring in the lungs from various insults such as infection, polluted air, and cigarette smoke. Spice extracts are also valuable for preventing such damage and, in fact, are significantly for this purpose more powerful than vitamins and minerals. Research at major labs proves that spice extracts are up to 20 times more powerful than the typical vitamin and/or mineral antioxidant.

While the vitamins and minerals are fairly potent antioxidants, natural plant chemicals may be regarded as super-potent. Numerous natural plant chemicals, such as phenols and flavonoids, have been shown to be up to 100 times more effective than vitamins or minerals. The ideal approach is to take a combination of antioxidant vitamins, minerals, and plant compounds in order to protect the lung tissue to the utmost. The fact is the lungs are direly in need of protection. Only natural compounds can achieve this.

Due to the destruction of the elastic walls of the lungs, as well as the alveoli, the ability of the lungs to expand and contract is severely compromised. Thus, the inability to expel inhaled air is one of the cardinal symptoms of emphysema. In essence once the air is inhaled, it becomes trapped within the lungs. Individuals with emphysema complain of shortness of breath and a feeling of suffocation. This trapping of air and suffocation makes emphysema one of the most gruesome of all diseases known.

Cigarette smoking is the primary cause of this condition. This type of smoke is so profoundly toxic to the lungs that it causes massive inflammation, leading to scarring and cellular breakdown. Immediately after inhalation, even the amount from a single puff results in cell damage. A single cigarette can destroy millions of cells. Plus, cigarette smoke destroys vitamins C and E, needed to keep the alveoli in optimal condition. A single cigarette destroys as much as 30 mg of vitamin C and 3 mg of vitamin E. A pack depletes virtually all of the vitamin C and E stores in the body. When these vitamins are depleted, these delicate air sacs degenerate, and, thus, they cannot properly deliver oxygen. The loss of these air sacs leads to disruption in the function of the entire body, since the body's ability to deliver oxygen to the blood is lost. If you smoke, quit. Otherwise, you risk permanent and irreversible lung damage and, certainly, premature death. However, all is not lost. This is because such smoke-induced damage can be largely reversed, that is through the intake of potent extracts of essential oils. It is the spice oils, that is oils of oregano, rosemary, sage, cloves, etc., which offer the most potent antioxidant and tissue-regenerative actions.

Treatment protocol

Take the antioxidant and antiseptic tonic, Oregacyn, 2 or more capsules twice daily. Also, rub oil of Oreganol and/or oil of rosemary on the chest at night. These oils may be added to a heavy fat, like coconut fat or cocoa butter, and rubbed onto the chest. Use the researched/tested Oreganol oil of oregano, which is 100% wild. Greek research determined that wild oregano may be up to 400% more powerful than the commercial type. The latter is often farm-raised, and the chemistry of farm-raised oregano is considerably different than that of the wild type. This certainly explains the difference in efficacy. The oil of oregano may also be taken internally, for instance, 3 to 5 drops twice daily under the tongue. Usually, the oil helps improve breathing dramatically. Avoid exposure to noxious fumes, especially cigarette smoke. Also, take selenium, 400 mcg daily and natural vitamin C (such as Flavin-C), about 500 mg or more daily. In order to speed healing or regeneration large amounts may be necessary. While synthetic vitamin C can upset the digestive tract, Flavin-C is completely non-toxic. It is well tolerated, even by those with sensitive digestive systems. In fact, it aids digestion. Plus, it is non-citrus. Furthermore, Flavin-C is exclusively from wild or natural sources and contains no ingredients from genetically engineered sources. For instance, virtually all synthetic vitamin C products are derived from corn sugars, and thus, they contain residues of genetically engineered components. These components may cause significant toxicity. In addition, take natural-source vitamin E, 400 to 800 I.U. daily as well as natural-source beta carotene, 50,000 I.U. daily. Bromazyme, a potent natural source of fruit enzymes, may aid in the dissolution of scar tissue as well as in the liberation from the lungs of toxins, particularly tar and particulate matter: take 3 capsules twice daily on an empty stomach.

Flu

Globally, this is the most common cause of infectious epidemics. It causes a greater amount of misery, as well as death, than any other episodic infectious disease.

The flu is an extremely dangerous illness, in fact, its dangers are often underestimated. *The Chicago Tribune*, September 2001, offers stark evidence for its potential for devastation. According to the *Tribune* in 1918 the flu killed 100 million people globally. People died quickly. No age group was immune but, surprisingly, 30 to 40 year old men, who would normally be resistant, were its primary victims. This is the pandemic that today's experts most greatly fear. The number of victims could be astronomical: perhaps several hundred million. However, the more likely scenario is that, globally, between 10 to 80 million will die, still an incredibly large number. In the recent past the powers of a new strain of flu were felt. In 1957 the Asian flu killed 70,000 Americans.

The flu normally lasts only about three days to a week. However, there has been developing a kind of increasing vulnerability to its toxicity. In certain instances the infection is lasting over ten days, which may indicate that there is a weakening of the populations' immunity. Incredibly, some victims suffer with it for nearly a month. Typically, the individual becomes exhausted and unable to function, suffering from aches, pains, nasal discharge and respiratory symptoms. Rarely, this leads to pneumonia, which may be fatal.

The source of the infection is usually contaminated air. Influenza spreads by droplets arising usually from human discharges. Sneezing and coughing liberate the virus on water droplets. It can live in this manner for at least 8 hours in the air. Thus, an epidemic is dependent upon the spread in civilized regions, where large numbers of people congregate. The original source is probably not man, but is, instead, swine. The virus flourishes in pig blood, and pigs excrete it in their urine, feces, and breath. Pork farms are the major site from which influenza spreads. This may explain why influenza often arises in China, where pig farms are common near populated regions.

The flu usually strikes suddenly. Symptoms can begin within 24 hours of exposure. It can spread fast. An entire family can succumb within hours. In fact, an entire community can succumb within days, perhaps hours. Thus, the medical facilities will be completely overwhelmed. The fact is modern medicine is incapable of offering any type of cure.

With the flu there is always a danger for a global epidemic, which occurs approximately once every 35 years. The world is overdue for a severe epidemic.

The history of the pandemics is revealing. They have occurred in 1510, 1557, 1580, 1593, 1658, 1675, 1729, 1762, 1780, 1788, 1830, 1846, 1857, 1889, and 1918. As 1918 was the last time a pandemic occurred, it is long overdue and will likely occur between 2003 and 2006, with the target year being

2005. When it occurs, it is possible that hundreds of thousands, perhaps millions, will die. Unless individuals are armed with the knowledge of potent natural cures, there will be little or no hope for survival.

If the pandemic type of flu strikes, all people are vulnerable. While it may not kill, long term damage can result. In severe cases complications develop. These complications include bacterial and fungal infections of the lungs, sinuses, ears, and mouth. Strep commonly attacks the weakened flu victim, as do molds and fungi. Thus, once the immune system is weakened by the flu virus the body is vulnerable to opportunistic infections. In some individuals a severe type of bronchitis may develop, which may last for several days and greatly weaken the individual. In rare instances pneumonia develops, which may lead to death. In pandemics fatal pneumonia occurs more frequently, causing a higher than usual death rate. The fact is influenza is one of the most dangerous of all infections, especially for the elderly. This year (2003) several children in England and America have suddenly died from flu-like symptoms. This is an ominous warning that a great flu pandemic is imminent.

The flu may so greatly compromise immunity that the individual may fail to completely recover, or it may take weeks or months to regain strength. Bizarre side effects can develop, including kidney damage, nerve damage, paralysis, numbness, pink eye, iritis, visual loss, oral blisters, shingles, nerve damage, and even baldness. In the extreme the virus may attack the brain, causing seemingly permanent neurological damage.

The human flu is spread by pigs. The 1918 flu was caused by a virus originating in swine, which mutated so that it could easily enter human cells. The pigs were immune, but humans had no immunity. Thus, the immune system was completely overwhelmed and failed to offer an adequate defense. Mark Gibbs of Australia's National University claims that researchers believe that the virus had infected pigs and then mutated, allowing it to aggressively invade humans.

Medically, there is nothing that can be done for the flu. The flu vaccine is virtually useless. The fact is there is no significant research proving efficacy or safety. Thus, it is largely an experimental therapy. What's more, it is fraught with side effects, including the serious paralytic condition known as Guillian-Barré syndrome. In this condition the vaccine causes damage to the spinal cord and brain, resulting in full body paralysis. It may also cause encephalitis, which has a high risk for fatality. Thus, the vaccine itself may cause permanent damage and/or death. The question is: does it truly prevent the flu? Are the positive benefits greater than the damage? The fact is any positive benefits have never been convincingly affirmed. Even if it were effective, supplies are unreliable. Furthermore, there is no guarantee that the proper type of vaccine or sufficient quantities thereof will be available to defend against the crisis. Plus, vaccines are invariably vulnerable to contamination with germs, as well as genetic material from germs, that is germ DNA. They may also contain unknown amounts of various chemical preservatives, including mercury, formaldehyde, synthetic phenol, and aluminum. Such chemicals are highly toxic to the immune system. According to Dr. H. Fudenberg, Ph.D., the mercury found in vaccines causes significant toxicity. For instance, he documented a ten-fold increased risk for Alzheimer's disease as a result of the flu shot. Certainly, the brain damage in this instance may be due to the mercury, but it could also be caused by an immune reaction against the brain.

Thus, it becomes readily apparent that the individual must learn about and utilize natural cures if he/she wishes "guaranteed survival." This is because only natural substances offer virus-killing powers without damaging the immune system or other organs.

The book *Microbiology and Man,* written in 1949, provides invaluable information about what the flu is and how it is caused. Influenza is described as an acute infection which strikes suddenly, lasting from one to seven days. The common symptoms haven't changed: achiness, fatigue, exhaustion, pains in the back and limbs, nasal discharge, and respiratory symptoms. Uncomplicated cases are usually mild, but they may greatly weaken the individual. This may lead to future disease or even a sudden bout of potentially fatal pneumonia. These early authors remind us that influenza may be elusive, that is the symptoms are so vague that it may not be correctly diagnosed. This may prove dangerous, because the flu must be taken seriously, and the proper treatment and precautions must be urgently administered.

The older theories regarding the cause of influenza are fascinating and are certainly accurate. The frank cause is a virus. However, early studies found that a bacteria is associated, the throat germ known as Hemophilus influenzae. This germ apparently contributes to the illness, but, obviously, the virus is the primary culprit. Apparently, the virus lives and reproduces in this bacteria.

The role of other germs, like Hemophilus, is exemplified by the infectious history in the main reservoir for the flu virus:

hogs. In Iowa in 1918 a disease appeared in hogs which was so similar to the human flu that it was promptly named "swine flu." The disease, which is exceedingly lethal, strikes a herd in the same way the flu virus strikes human groups. In 1931 Richard Shope of the Rockefeller Institute in a series of well designed investigations in pigs showed that the disease was due to a virus and that a bacteria, the Hemophilus influenza, was also a contributor. Dr. Shope found that it was necessary for the germs to be present simultaneously to cause severe flu.

This is how the virus and bacteria, at least in hogs, are related. Swine flu usually only occurs from October to December. Shope found that the Hemophilus germ, which is needed to produce the disease in hogs, was present all year, primarily in the nasal and respiratory passages. In contrast, the virus is only in swine seasonally. Since viruses cannot survive without infecting, that is parasitizing, cells, they are rarely permanent residents and are usually cleared by the immune system, or they may enter into a form of hibernation. Shope was originally unable to determine where the virus went in the remaining months, in other words, it couldn't just appear out of nowhere. It had to have a host. He suspected that there must be another agent, a parasite, which keeps the virus viable. He found two such parasites, both of them worms. One was the hog lungworm, and the other, incredibly, was the common earthworm. This is how transmission and infectivity are maintained. During the acute flu infection the hog lungworm becomes infected with the virus. These worms are coughed up, swallowed, and excreted in the feces. The residue in the feces is eaten by the earthworm, which acts as a host. In other words, the eggs of the hog worm actually hatch within the earthworm, living off of it. The hog then eats the earthworms, and the cycle continues endlessly. When the earthworms are digested, the lungworm's eggs, infected with flu virus, are liberated, ultimately reaching the lungs, where they develop into worms. Yet, this is insufficient to provoke severe flu, that is unless the bacteria, Hemophilus influenza (swine variety), is present. Thus, the hog, laden with various parasites, harbors and maintains the very germ which has the potential of causing millions of deaths globally. This may in part explain the scriptural prohibition against the eating or raising of pork.

Treatment protocol

For mild cases take the multi-spice antiseptic formula, that is the Oregacyn, 2 capsules three times daily (with meals). For tough cases take it more often, as much as a capsule or two every hour. Note: while Oregacyn, a spice extract, is safe, excessive intake has a possible side effect: constipation. This is due to the destruction of the normal healthy intestinal bacteria. The intestinal bacteria account for a large bulk of the stool. To correct this take large amounts of healthy bacteria (as supplements), or eat large quantities of yogurt. As a potent preventive agent Oregacyn may be used in small doses: take one or two capsules daily. For additional power take the oil of wild oregano (Oreganol), 2 to 5 drops under the tongue several times daily. Continue until symptoms disappear. For tough cases the key is rapidity; it may be necessary to take it every few minutes until symptoms clear. Oil of wild oregano is an absolute cure for influenza. What's more, Oregacyn is highly antiviral. If a sufficient amount is taken, it will destroy the flu virus. Avoid the consumption of pork, including ham, bacon, sausage, pepperoni, bologna, bratwursts, hot dogs, etc. Also, do not eat or drink food containing refined sugar.

Hay fever

This is one of the most commonly occurring of all allergic diseases, afflicting tens of millions of North Americans. It mainly attacks the nose and eyes, causing congestion, sneezing, and nasal drainage.

The term hay fever is misleading. Usually, there is no fever. Plus, hay is only one of many hundreds of protein/pollen sources which may provoke it. However, the "hay" portion of the name is revealing: wet hay is a source of various pollens, as well as molds, and reactions to it by farmers and other individuals working closely with hay may have initiated the name. The fact is wet hay breeds molds, and these molds produced untold billions of spores, which may be liberated in hot or windy weather. Thus, a more correct name would be moldy hay fever.

Hay fever can cause a great deal of misery, even though it is not serious. However, the discomfort, which includes obstructed breathing, sneezing, watery eyes, itching of the eyes/nose, and nasal discharge, is serious, since it significantly affects lifestyle.

Hay fever is usually most severe during August and September, finally ending at the first frost. The fact that it ends at this time is a clear indication of the role of molds as a major cause, since cold weather destroys them. There is also a spring type due to tree pollens and the pollens of certain grasses. Yet, mold counts are also high at this time. Obviously, the risks are greatest when the pollen and mold counts are high. Thus, the symptoms of hay fever are due to a reaction against both pollens and molds. However, at the root of this is a rarely recognized fact, that is that there may be an underlying chronic sinus or lung infection, which makes the individual more vulnerable to the hay fever allergens. Mold/yeast infestation is the usual cause of this undiagnosed infection. In other words, the prior existence of molds, yeasts, and other germs within the sinuses and respiratory tract create the vulnerability. When the mold counts in the air rise, such individuals may react violently.

Pollen is an outdoor substance; the counts indoors are comparatively low. Staying indoors in an air conditioned home is one rather extreme, in fact, impractical therapy. Pollen counts are also low in the mountains or seaside. Incredibly, there is no truly pollen-free region, except, perhaps, the far north of Canada. Even so, doctors may recommend that a sufferer visit the seaside or the high mountains as a therapy. What's more, the seashore offers relief only when the wind is blowing in from the ocean. However, this is a rather extreme therapy. Fortunately, there is a solution for correcting this distressing condition without leaving your home.

The medical treatment for hay fever is essentially nonexistent. There are no drugs which cure it, only a few, such as antihistamines, modify symptoms. A specialized therapy known as "desensitization" may be offered. However, this is both painful and cumbersome and only occasionally offers a cure. Thus, natural remedies are the only solutions.

Treatment protocol

Crude extracts of wild medicinal spices offer significant anti-histaminic and anti-mold actions. Spice and herb extracts offer safety unavailable from over-the-counter agents.

Certain spice extracts, notably oil of oregano, clove, sage, and bay leaf, offer potent antihistaminic actions. In this function they are highly aggressive, that is they are fast-acting. What's more, they exhibit significant antifungal powers. Thus, they are the ideal tonics for reversing this condition. Also, oil of wild oregano, taken under the tongue, can be an effective treatment for rapidly halting the symptoms of this condition. To reverse hayfever take Oregacyn, which contains multiple antihistaminic spices, one or two capsules as needed. This is so potent that it can be deemed a total cure for this condition. Also, take oil of wild oregano, a few drops under the tongue as needed. Natural vitamin C is antihistaminic; take Flavin-C, three capsules twice or more daily. Avoid the intake of commercial antihistamines, especially nasal sprays. The latter cause damage to the delicate nasal passages, increasing the risks for chronic sinus and/or nasal disorders. Nasal sprays are a primary cause of chronic sinus infections.

Histoplasmosis

This is a rather serious lung infection caused by a fungus. This type of fungus most commonly grows in moist climates, especially in river valleys. Areas where birds congregate are another hot spot, because bird droppings cause the fungus to flourish. In the Ohio and Mississippi river valleys the infection is common. Thousands, perhaps millions, of people may harbor the infection and be unaware of it. Incredibly, according to the National Tuberculosis and Respiratory Disease Association as many as 50 million Americans unknowingly suffer from histoplasmosis. That amount was based upon old research. A more reasonable estimate is that histoplasmosis affects some 90 million Americans. That is nearly one of three individuals.

Children are particularly vulnerable to this infection and for some unknown reason males are more commonly affected than females. In fact, the ratio is nearly seven to one. In the Midwest there are millions of males who unknowingly suffer the infection. The common Midwestern "summer/fall flu" may, in fact, be a fungal infection in the form of histoplasmosis. The only difference between it and the flu is that histoplasmosis may last for weeks, and it may take weeks or months to recover. Chest X-rays may reveal that what was presumed to be the flu is instead a persistent fungal lung infection. However, even if the chest X-rays are negative this fails to rule out histoplasmosis, since in its early stages medical testing may be equivocal.

The fungus attacks the lymphatic system, as well as the liver and spleen, causing enlargement of these organs. However, the lungs suffer the brunt of the damage, and this is how doctors usually discover it, that is they see evidence of it on X-ray.

Histoplasmosis is an aggressive organism. It attacks a wide range of organs, particularly the liver, spleen, lungs, lymph nodes, bone marrow, adrenals, and intestines. It even invades the white blood cells and may thereby evade the immune system. The fungus is an aggressive pathogen, capable of digesting human tissue. This is because it produces a wide range of digestive enzymes, which break down human protein, accelerating its invasive abilities. For the condition to be cured the fungus must be utterly destroyed. Spice extracts, which are highly antifungal, offer the best hope for a cure.

Treatment protocol

Take a multiple-spice extract, such as Oregacyn, 2 or 3 capsules twice daily. Take also Oreganol, 10 drops under the tongue twice daily. To further cleanse the lungs of pathogens and improve blood flow to the lungs take Respira Clenz, 10 to 20 drops twice daily. Also, increase the intake of foods rich in essential fatty acids. The essential fatty acids strengthen immunity and help increase the resistance against fungal infections. Take primrose oil, 6 capsules twice daily. Selenium is protective against lung fungal infections. The regular intake of this mineral assists the immune system in preventing the colonization by fungi. Take organically bound selenium, about 400 mcg daily. Note: Sodium selenite is potentially toxic. Use only organically bound type of selenium such as selenium thiamine and/or selenium yeast.

Mold spore infection

Mold spores readily enter the respiratory tract. This region is the ideal region for their growth. It is warm, moist, and cool. This is the type of environment in which molds thrive. This may explain why medical researchers are discovering that virtually all humans suffer some degree of mold or fungal infestation. According to the New York Times doctors have proven that even supposedly healthy individuals have bizarre fungi growing in their tissues, particularly within their respiratory tracts. The area of greatest infestation is apparently the sinuses. Researchers have found mold-related, tentacle-producing fungi in the sinuses of "virtually everyone", including species such as Penicillium, Bipolaris, Cladosporium, and Alternaria. None of these are normal inhabitants of the respiratory system. According to a study done at the Mayo Clinic the immune system regards such fungi as irritants and makes every attempt to destroy them. In other words, they are all invaders. Yet, the immune system may fail to kill them, as fungi have evolved an immense capacity to invade and survive. There are no drugs which can kill these fungi. Natural substances are the only solution.

Treatment protocol

Molds (and fungi) readily attack the sinuses, causing pain, swelling, mucus build-up, and inflammation. They cause blockage, preventing the flow of naturally-produced sinus fluids. This causes a major disruption in function, since the sinus fluids are needed to wash poisons and microbes from the respiratory canals. Thus, it is crucial to destroy invasive molds and fungi to achieve optimal health. Wild oregano and similar pungent spices are the most potent mold killers known. Take Oregacyn, one or more capsules two or three times daily with food. Take also oil of wild oregano (P73), five or more drops under the tongue twice daily. For tough conditions increase the dose, for instance, 10 to 20 drops two or three times daily. Vitamin A is required to maintain healthy mucous membranes in order to prevent fungal invasion. As a vitamin A source eat a can or two of sardines daily. Also, eat organic calf's or lamb's liver at least twice weekly. Take a natural vitamin A supplement, 10,000 I.U. daily.

Nasal polyps

This condition is caused by the hypertrophy of the mucous

membranes of the lining of the nose. According to *Dorland's Medical Dictionary* nasal polyps are a type of tumor.

Nasal polyps are evidence of the existence of irritants. The irritants may be chemical or microbial. For instance, viral infections may induce them. What's more, they are a sign of nutritional imbalances. Deficiencies of vitamins A and C have been associated with the development of polyps. In fact, some texts describe them as a deliberate sign of vitamin A deficiency. The deficiency of these vitamins as a cause makes sense, because they are both needed to protect the mucous membranes against toxicity as well as viral infection.

Nasal polyps can become sufficient in size to obstruct breathing. In this respect they can prove dangerous. Polyps may also develop as a consequence of drug therapy. Despite this drugs are the common treatment. Yet, since the polyps are caused largely by nutritional deficiency, as well as viral infection, the drugs fail to treat the cause and, thus, usually fail to correct it.

Treatment should include a diet high in vitamin A- and C-rich foods. Ideal food sources of vitamin A include organic liver, squash, sweet potatoes, sardines, salmon, egg yolk, and dark green leafy vegetables. Excellent sources of natural vitamin C include citrus fruit, guava, papaya, kiwi, citrus juice, lemons, limes, unsweetened currant juice, spinach, and broccoli. Refined sugar and flour should be completely avoided. All alcoholic beverages must be avoided. If you smoke, quit.

Treatment protocol

As a vitamin A source eat a can or two of sardines daily. Also, eat organic calf's or lamb's liver at least twice weekly. Take oil of wild oregano, five drops sublingually twice daily. Also, take

Oregacyn, one or two capsules twice daily. For severe cases take larger amounts such as two to four capsules twice daily. As a source of crude unprocessed natural vitamin C take Flavin-C, three capsules twice daily. Flavin-C contains anti-inflammatory bioflavonoids, which help decrease the swelling of the polyps and prevent recurrence. Also, take a vitamin A supplement, about 10,000 I.U. daily.

Pleurisy

This pneumonia-like condition is due to inflammation of the linings of the lungs, that is the pleura. It often occurs as a secondary effect to pneumonia. It may also be a sign of tuberculosis. The fact is a sudden case of pleurisy where no other cause is obvious often warns of hidden TB.

In this condition the individual is afflicted with the sudden onset of a very sharp pain, like a stabbing pain. The pain occurs with every breath. Coughing causes severe stabbing pain. Usually, there is high fever and chills as well as aches and pains. Bacteria are a primary cause, but fungi and molds can also provoke it. So can parasites, which may invade the pleural membranes.

Bacteria can cause severe inflammation, leading to scar formation. The inflammation and scarring causes the pleuritic pain. Treatment should be aimed not only at eradicating the germs but also at the reversal of the inflammation, plus the breakdown of the scarring.

Treatment protocol

Bacteria and molds, the major causes of pleurisy, quickly succumb to the powers of multiple spice extracts. Certain of the extracts, such as extracts of wild oregano and cloves, exhibit significant pain-killing powers. Take Oregacyn, the multiple edible spice extract, 2 capsules three or more times daily. Also, take a few extra capsules whenever the pain strikes. Rub P73 oil of wild oregano over the ribs and on the mid-back as often as necessary. Take 2 or more drops of the oil under the tongue two or more times daily. To digest the scars and reduce inflammation take the protein-digesting plant enzymes concentrate, that is Bromazyme, 3 or 4 capsules twice daily on an empty stomach. Also, take the anti-inflammatory citrus bioflavonoid complex, Flavin-C, 4 or more capsules twice daily on an empty stomach.

Hot tea can help relieve the pain, especially if hot spices are added. Chop or slice fresh ginger root, and add to your favorite hot herbal tea. Clove buds may also be added. Drink several cups daily.

Pneumonia

This is perhaps the most serious of all respiratory illnesses. Virtually any type of germ can cause it. Often, it is caused by a particular bacteria, known descriptively as pneumococcus. This germ normally lives in the nose, sinuses, and throat. If it does get into the lungs, in the normal individual it is rapidly destroyed. However, if the immune system is compromised, the germ may overgrow, causing severe infection and inflammation. This most commonly occurs in the weak and debilitated. Hospitalized patients, especially those with cancer or AIDS, are the most vulnerable to developing this serious disease. In fact, pneumonia is the primary cause of death in these individuals.

There are numerous types of pneumonia. These types may be caused by a wide range of germs, including various bacteria as well as viruses, yeasts, molds, and parasites. This is why the diagnosis of pneumonia, that is which microbe is responsible, is often so elusive. Medically, for proper treatment to be dispensed the exact cause must be known. Otherwise, the wrong medicine may be given. This may, in fact, aggravate the illness.

Pneumonia is often a secondary effect of other conditions. For instance, let's say an elderly but healthy person has a hip fracture. This results in stress and immobility. The individual is hospitalized in a weakened state. Hospital food is notoriously of poor quality, which further compromises resistance. Thus, the patient's condition continues to deteriorate. Pneumonia develops and often kills the individual. Hospitalized cancer patients are also particularly vulnerable. Their resistance is compromised, plus they often undergo toxic therapies, such as radiation or chemotherapy, which greatly depress immunity. When the powers of the immune system decline, which is the ultimate consequence of such toxic therapies, the lungs are readily colonized by a host of pathogens such as Candida albicans, pneumococcus, staph, E. coli, molds, and/or various parasites. As a result, the individual rapidly succumbs. In such weakened individuals infection by noxious germs readily develops: the germs multiply unchecked. There are no drugs to treat such infections. The only hope in the hospital environment is the patient's own resistance.

Drug-resistant highly pathogenic germs abound in hospital environments. The air ducts and room air are fully contaminated. Patients inhale the germs, which may rapidly infect them. Tuberculosis may also be spread in this manner. These germs aggressively attack the body, causing life-threatening infections. There is far less risk for fatal pneumonia in cancer patients treated outside the hospital than those treated within it.

Hospitals house a vast number of pathogens, many of which are highly virulent. The fact is such germs are freaks of nature. These biochemical freaks are the consequence of the overuse of antibiotics and are known medically as mutant bacteria. The mutants cause frighteningly severe infections, which rapidly induce fatalities, plus there are no medical cures against them. Recently (March 2003), a new and highly infectious type of pneumonia was recognized. Known as "atypical" pneumonia this is probably due to a virus, although the exact cause has yet to be determined. Outbreaks of atypical pneumonia occur yearly. Often, the source of the outbreaks is animal viruses. The most likely animal reservoir is poultry or swine. However, ultimately, the viruses mutate, infecting humans. There are no possible vaccines or drugs for such infections. Here, natural medicines are the only possible cures.

A deadly type of atypical pneumonia has recently developed. Known as SARS (Severe Acute Respiratory Syndrome) it was first discovered in early 2003 and is wreaking havoc throughout the world. Southeast Asia is suffering the greatest degree of damage, although SARS could readily disrupt any region. In southeast Asia hundreds of people have died and thousands have been hospitalized, many in intensive care. Hospital care workers are particularly victimized. As they became sickened they spread the infection among the public. This type of pneumonia, like many others, is disseminated through close contact, via coughing and sneezing. However, people at considerable distance have also been infected. Yet, anyone in close proximity to a SARS victim will readily contract this disease. As indicated by the name SARS is particularly aggressive: even young vital adults, as well as athletes, may succumb. The scope of this dilemma is denoted by the *Financial Times*, March 2003, which calls this germ a "virulent" cause of a global epidemic.

The symptoms of this condition are similar to the flu but more severe. However, the effects on the lungs are dissimilar. In SARS there is significant breathing difficulty, shortness of breath, and even wheezing, which are rarely seen in flu. The fact is in SARS people simply cannot breathe. Plus, they are debilitated by a deep dry unrelenting cough. In contrast, the flu makes people sick, but rarely causes pneumonia, that is except in its global pandemic form. Other symptoms of SARS include high fever, chills, dry cough, lack of appetite, headache, and malaise. A key symptom is a dry racking cough, which arises deep from the lungs. The fact is a deep dry cough combined with a fever is virtually an assurance of the diagnosis. Diarrhea may also occur.

Often, SARS begins merely as a type of flu with muscle aches, fever, and a dry cough. As it progresses, the infection lodges in the lower lungs, causing breathing difficulty. The progression toward a serious illness is often rapid: within hours physical collapse may occur. The virus may also attack the linings of the lungs and the sinuses, causing congestion and bleeding. This bleeding is a serious sign of damage to the internal organs. The fact is this germ, if unchecked, causes massive lung damage, some reports indicating it even dissolves lung tissue. No organ is immune from its aggression. Autopsies on SARS victims discovered evidence of bleeding of the internal organs, an ominous sign of the destructive and invasive powers of this virus.

The exact cause of this syndrome remains elusive. However, the majority of research implicates certain viruses, notably paramyxoviruses and coronaviruses. While most researchers point to the coronavirus family it could be a combination of both. These viruses are aggressive respiratory pathogens. Such viruses readily attack and destroy human cells, including the cells lining the respiratory passages. Apparently, these viruses attach to the lung cells, ultimately killing them. The fact is while researchers have been concerned about the return of a killer flu SARS behaves like a killer cold. So says Nigel Hawker in the *London Times*, who writes that a "killer cold" is a syndrome of the worst kind, because "as everyone knows colds are easily spread and have no (medical) cure (parentheses mine)."

The virus responsible for SARS is highly infective. Medically, nothing can be done to stop it from infecting the tissues. The aggressive nature of this germ is due to the fact that it was in all likelihood originally a porcine virus. In other words, it is an animal virus, which has mutated to infect humans. Hogs serve as the reservoir. Think about it. If such a germ is tough enough to sicken or kill hogs, what could it do to humans? The fact is such hog-derived viruses are highly invasive and may quickly decimate the individual. Hog and human DNA are highly similar. Thus, hog viruses can quickly mutate into a human form. To halt this epidemic the hogs in the area of origin should be slaughtered.

While killer flus also originate from hogs, the SARS virus has proven equally diabolical. The fact is virtually half of all exposed individuals develop the infection in the form of life-threatening pneumonia. Here, the lungs become utterly infected, filling with fluid, germs, and pus. As many as 15% die, although some experts claim the death rate as high as 50%. The prestigious medical journal, the *Lancet*, claims a death rate in people over the age of 60 as high as 55%. What's more, those who do survive often fair poorly. A high percentage of survivors suffer permanent lung damage. This damage can include permanent scarring of the lungs.

Globally, authorities have taken this epidemic seriously. At the time of this publication it has developed into a virulent pandemic, creating intense fear and pandemonium. The germ is spread readily through close contact. It is also airborne, meaning it can infect individuals at some distance. During April 2003 in Hong Kong an entire high rise became contaminated, with some 300 residents infected. Here, researchers are unsure whether the spread was airborne or via direct contact. What's more, the SARS virus readily spreads in airplanes. Ultimately, investigators determined that, indeed, it was airborne, that is it spread through the exhaust fans of restrooms. In another case it spread throughout an Air China jet, sickening dozens of passengers. Thus, the SARS virus may be readily spread through the air, in these cases through the air ducts and vents of high rises and jet airliners. Incredibly, the 300 Hong Kong residents were moved from their homes to high security isolation camps. The world is not prepared for this. Thus, a major catastrophe is likely. Once it contaminates an object it remains infective for up to 48 hours.

The SARS virus is highly virulent, perhaps one of the most life-threatening viruses every known. If it mutates into even more virulent forms, it could cause a highly fatal global pandemic.

In Hong Kong airports and airlines were barring sick passengers. Schools and even hospitals have been closed. In Toronto, Canada, where officials have taken this epidemic with utmost seriousness, numerous hospitals have been closed and over a thousand potentially exposed individuals were quarantined. Here, in less than a month more than twenty people died.

In April 2003 the situation in Hong Kong was regarded as dire. H. Yeoung, president of Hong Kong's Doctor's Union, claims the circumstance to be so dangerous that in Hong Kong "everyone should wear surgical masks and all schools must be shut for two weeks." Also, in Canada paramedics exposed to the germ were quarantined.

Once the germ is disseminated, it remains infective for days. Entire rooms and buildings can become hopelessly contaminated. Plus, again, the fact is no one knows for sure the cause. This illustrates the importance of utilizing natural germicides, as well as natural virus killers, as the preferred treatment. This is because a wide range of natural compounds effectively kills viruses plus a host of other germs. What's more, they are non-toxic, so they can be taken/applied in large doses at the needed frequency. They can be used aggressively even in the highly vulnerable, like newborns, infants, children, the immune compromised, and the elderly.

Currently, SARS is virtually everywhere, although the hotbed of infection is southeast Asia. In addition to China and Hong Kong, where untold thousands are infected, cases have been reported in Singapore, Malaysia, Vietnam, Taiwan, Indonesia, Australia, South Africa, Thailand, Philippines, England, Romania, Bulgaria, Germany, France, Spain, Italy, Brazil, Mongolia, New Zealand, South Korea, Kuwait, Switzerland, Ireland, Canada, and the United States.

In the fight against this disease there are two natural medicines to rely upon: Germ-a-Clenz and Oregacyn. The latter is the front line of defense. It is a powerful germ killer, truly life-saving. It may be taken preventatively: one capsule twice daily. If exposed or sickened, it should be taken aggressively, like two or more capsules three times daily. In severe cases it can be taken even more aggressively, like 2 to 4 capsules several times daily, or even every other hour (Note: be sure to take it with food, juice or with plenty of water). The Germ-a-Clenz is the ideal air sterilizer. Use it preventatively in all possible scenarios. Simply spray it high in the air in any room or region that may be contaminated. Spray in a tissue and breathe, or spray it directly into the mouth and/or nose. Use it for prevention in any area where people congregate. Keep both the Germ-a-Clenz and Oregacyn available at all times. Always have it available in the car, office, or other strategic places. Never go anywhere without it. The point is when an individual contracts SARS if at least he or she takes Oregacyn, premature death will be prevented. The Germ-a-Clenz can also prevent it, that is by destroying the germ in the air or on surfaces. It also makes a super throat spray. For best results spray it repeatedly at the roof of the mouth.

Oregacyn will neutralize the SARS virus. Germ-a-Clenz can neutralize its airborne components. Both of these potent natural medicines should be used aggressively. They aggressively make the difference, that is between survival or death. Plus, they can save the lives of friends, loved ones, and even total strangers. Thus, to halt the onslaught of future epidemics natural medicines, notably the Oregacyn and Germ-a-Clenz, as well as oil of wild oregano, must be relied upon. In fact, they must be the absolute treatment of choice. In preliminary trials natural medicines have recently been shown to be equal in efficacy to drugs, plus the majority of such medicines are free from serious side effects. This is a blessing from a power which is greater than humans. Amazingly, it is the divinely-ordained remedies which are saving lives, not the synthetics, that is man-made, ones. In other words, the components of oil of wild oregano as well as Oregacyn—various wild spices—are made by a power beyond comprehension, that is almighty God.

In truly severe SARS the Oregacyn may be used super-aggressively, like several capsules every hour. Also, use oil of wild oregano, rubbing it into the chest, back, and feet, as well as taking it under the tongue. Use also the Super Strength oil of oregano. It is effective as a topical rub and can also be taken sublingually for a direct effect.

In the view of some "experts" SARS is not as dire as many might believe. They claim that it is far from the type of diaboli-cal killer they have been expecting to strike humanity, like the 1918 flu, which killed millions. However, such an attitude of minimizing the risks is itself dangerous. If a casual approach is taken by top officials and the public fails to take the appropriate precautions, this itself will greatly increase the risks. Proper action must be taken immediately. Otherwise, SARS could become a brutal global epidemic, eventually killing thousands, even millions. Every effort must be taken to halt the spread of the disease. Otherwise, deaths which are potentially preventable will occur. The fact is at the time of this publication SARS has killed hundreds of individuals, sickening thousands of others. In China, where the epidemic is out of control, tens of thousands could be killed. Normal healthy adults have succumbed to it, as have chil-dren. None of these people were sick prior. Thus, this disease is a serious and diabolical killer.

The consensus is that SARS is an animal virus, which has

mutated to infect humans. No one can be sure of the original animal reservoir. It is likely from pigs, but considering the source of the outbreak, that is southern China, virtually any animal could be the source, including chickens, ducks, cows, cats, dogs: even rats. In fact, in southern China many people eat a wide range of carnivorous animals, such as dogs, wild pigeons, birds of prey, and cats—even rats—regarding them as delicacies. Such dire habits are likely the origin of the infection. This is because the flesh of such animals, all of which are carnivores, is highly contaminated with microbes. These microbes cannot be fully killed by cooking. Thus, the carnivore-derived germs infect the cells of the eater, where they reproduce. There, they adopt the genetic structure of human cells, making them highly virulent. The infected human acts essentially like the viruses' synthetic factory, where they reproduce by the billions. In other words, they adapt to the human genetic code, parasitizing it. This means that the infection, rather than originating from airborne spread, such as from a pig's breath to a human's lungs, could be the result of highly destructive hygienic or dietary habits, that is the eating of the flesh of contaminated carnivores. Unless such practices are curbed, global epidemics of such a dire nature, true killers of humanity, will continue to develop, destroying much of the human race. In essence, SARS is a type of human plague that may have originated from contaminated animals such as pigs, ducks, rats, or wild game.

Speculation exists that SARS stems from a genetically engineered, that is man-made, virus. However, evidence proving it is lacking. This thinking is based upon the fact that the virus contains genetic material from a variety of animals, including mice, poultry, and pigs. Yet, it is equally plausible that aberrant genetic material arises from natural genetic alterations. For instance, exotic cats, which are eaten in China, prey on mice. Virus particles from mouse viruses could easily be incorporated into feline viruses. Thus, nature creates a genetic mix. This might explain the incorporation of mouse genetic material observed in the suspected SARS virus. The fact is the SARS virus behaves like a virus from a carnivorous animal. This would explain its incredibly aggressive and destructive behavior. This must be considered the source until proven otherwise. The fact is just as this book was going to press such a link was discovered. According to the *Chicago Tribune*, May 24, 2003, researchers in Hong Kong found evidence of SARS-like viruses in various "exotic" mammals, including a wild cat and raccoon-like dog. Further proof for such a connection is the fact that more than 30% of the early SARS cases from Guangdong occurred among food handlers, including those who sell such carnivorous animals. This is virtually certain proof that unnatural dietary habits are the cause of this pandemic.

It was the Prophet Muhammad who first delineated the harmful consequences of aberrant dietary habits. He categorically prohibited the consumption of the flesh of carnivores, including pigs. Through his rulings the flesh of dogs, cats, and similar carnivorous creatures were clearly established as unfit for human consumption. This is little surprise to true followers of scripture, who are aware of such prohibitions, that is from the Old Testament. Ultimately, such prohibitions are merely common sense. Anyone who observes the dietary and hygienic habits of such creatures must conclude they are inedible. Obviously, as is demonstrated by the current experience, that is the SARS epidemic, these prohibitions are strictly for one purpose: the protection of the health of the human race. Certainly, in the past such unhealthy dietary habits have led to killer epidemics.

The actual cause of SARS has yet to be proven definitively. Certainly, it is a type of virus. Yet, what is definite is that there is no medical treatment. Antibiotics are useless, in fact, counterproductive. Now, it is being shown that a number of germs may be the cause, that is there may be several viruses. This illustrates the value of natural substances, which are capable of killing a wide range of germs. Spice extracts are the most potent of these. A variety of studies proves that such extracts kill a wide range of germs, in some cases, all germs known. A study by Siddiqui in *Medical Science Research* is revealing. Here, spice extracts, such as those used in Oregacyn and Germ-a-Clenz, killed all viruses tested on contact. The researchers were so amazed that they described the spices' destructive actions as "remarkable". The fact is the spice oils essentially disintegrated the viruses, even difficult-to-kill ones such as herpes. Thus, spice extracts offer the potential to cure a wide range of the plagues of modern humankind, including SARS. What's more, SARS has no medical cure. Spice extracts, such as the components of Oregacyn, have been shown to kill coronaviruses in test tubes. This is why spice extracts, such as Oreganol and Oregacyn, are ideal. As an alternative to antibiotics, which are useless for this condition, a highly aggressive approach might be necessary such as taking a few capsules every half hour or every hour combined with the spice oils taken sublingually.

Such aggressive therapy makes sense. Once the SARS viruses overtake the cells' genetic machinery, they reproduce by the billions, in fact, tens of billions, every hour. Within 24 hours of the original infection literally trillions of viruses may be produced within the body. An utterly potent approach must be administered to halt such an attack. Thus, the counterattack must be stronger than the viral attack. Only spice extracts offer such potent aggression. Siddiqui says they disintegrate viruses on contact. This has certainly been my experience, that is with highly sick humans. I have observed that spice extracts save lives, even reversing potentially fatal types of pneumonia. I have noticed that such extracts halt symptoms, even full fledged infections, within hours—even minutes.

Certain dietary restrictions may be necessary to curb this epidemic. Certainly, the intake of pork or pork products must be halted. During the epidemic the intake of commercial chicken or duck in the epidemic area may need to be restricted. Ultimately, it is advisable to switch from commercial chicken/duck to organic or farm-raised types. Also, avoid the consumption of foods which suppress the immune system such as sweets, white flour products, refined vegetable oils, deep fried oils, nitrated/processed meats, and, of course, refined sugar. Drugs which weaken immunity must also be avoided, particularly aspirin, ibuprofen, cortisone (including prednisone), and antibiotics.

Yet, ultimately, a medicinal approach is required, that is the intake of powerful natural substances which work. Oregacyn is one such a substance. The potent effects of Oregacyn are recorded by the documented case histories:

Case History 1: In the United States in late February 2003, a woman developed a bizarre syndrome soon after departing a commercial flight. Her symptoms included terrible muscle aches, deep dry cough, high temperature, and total exhaustion. It appeared to be a SARS-like syndrome. I personally cared for the person, who was exceptionally ill. Immediately, she took Oregacyn, about 2 to 4 capsules every few hours. As the infection progressed she coughed up large amounts of blood-speckled mucus. Within three days her fever broke and she was fully functional. This was a dramatic improvement for a medically incurable syndrome. Further treatment cured the lingering deep cough, which was eliminated within 10 days.

Case History 2: In April 2003, a woman, after flying from Spain to London, developed unusual respiratory symptoms. As a medical practitioner she found the symptoms to be highly strange. Virtually every time she would breathe she coughed. It was a dry non-productive cough. She also suffered from a constricted sensation in the chest. Two Oregacyn were given. Within 10 minutes the cough was eliminated, never to return. She was able to breathe freely. What's more, she mentioned that she had never before experienced such a dramatic reversal of such severe symptoms.

SARS is beyond dangerous. It is beyond an epidemic. The fact is it is precisely a repeat of the 1918 pandemic. Like the latter, if unchecked, it will surely kill tens of thousands, even millions. The only hope for reversing it is aggressive use of natural substances capable of killing viruses such as wild spice extracts.

Treatment protocol

For pneumonia in general plenty of rest is necessary. The room should be quiet: no television or radio should be allowed. Soft music may be played, however, quiet time is superior for healing. Back rubs and massages are helpful. Anyone entering the room must wash the hands before touching the victim. Also, the hands must be washed thoroughly after touching. Then, spray them with Germ-a-Clenz. Drink freshly squeezed grapefruit or orange juice. Coffee and black tea should be avoided. Chocolate and sugar should also be avoided. The diet should be free of all milk products, particularly cheese. Little food should be eaten. For nourishment clear beef or chicken broth soups are ideal. During severe infections heavy meals rich in protein interfere with the healing process.

The air must be cleansed with essential oils. In a spray bottle add hot water along with antiseptic essential oils. Or, use the Germ-a-Clenz pump spray. This spray is so potent that it completely sterilizes the room. Shake well and pump spray the room. Spray any bedding and upholstery. Do this by spraying high in the air and allowing the mist to drift down upon it. Repeat several times daily as aggressively as necessary until the condition is resolved. This spray is highly effective. It will make an enormous difference in the condition, because it purifies the air. The most potent herbal tonic is Oregacyn, two or more capsules three times daily. For severe cases take it more frequently, as well as in larger doses, even as much as two to four caps every hour. In dire circumstances take it every half-hour, as much as 4 to 6 capsules per dose. If possible, be sure to take such high doses with food or juice. The point is be aggressive, that is as aggressive as necessary to halt the infection. Also, take oil of wild Oreganol oil, 10 or more drops several times daily (the Oreganol is edible and safe to take in large amounts). For severe cases take it more often, like every hour or even every half hour. Also, rub the oil on the feet several times daily until the fever breaks. The oil may also be rubbed spine as well as over the lung reflexes. Raw potent tonic. Eat as much raw honey as poss a day. The best medicinal raw hone Mediterranean. Excellent types include wild oreg thistle honey. These honeys are only available via mail order. To order call 1-800-243-5242. In Canada call 1-905-634-9480. These types of crude raw honeys are safe for all ages, even infants.

Onions are also a potent antiviral remedy. The juice of raw onions reliably kills any virus. Simply juice several onions. Add parsley juice to modify the taste. Drink a quarter cup as often as needed until symptoms are eliminated. I used this juice to obliterate a SARS-like syndrome in a respiratory therapist.

Rhinitis (runny nose)

This is more correctly described as a symptom rather than a disease. The question is what is causing such voluminous nasal and/or sinus irritation? Studies at Mayo Clinic indicate that fungal infection is the primary cause. Other factors include mite dust sensitivity or even mite infection. Pollen allergy also plays a role.

Rhinitis is an exceptionally common problem and a major cause of disability. There is nothing more miserable than a constantly running or inflamed nose.

Treatment protocol

Fungal infection is the most likely cause of rhinitis. Currently, the type of fungus is unknown, but there may be dozens of

...es. The fact that fungal infection is the obvious cause comes readily evident by the fact that all known treatments for this condition, including antibiotics, cortisone, and nasal sprays, fail to resolve it. In contrast, natural antifungal agents, such as oil of wild oregano and, particularly, Oregacyn multiple spice extract, are potent and rapid cures for this condition. To reverse rhinitis take Oreganol oil of wild oregano, five or more drops several times daily under the tongue. Continue this dosage until the symptoms are resolved. Also, take Oregacyn, one or more capsules twice daily with food. Avoid the use of commercial antihistamines, particularly nasal sprays. If used chronically, the latter cause damage to the delicate nasal and sinus membranes, which perpetuates this condition. Also, make a radical change in the diet. Avoid processed foods, refined sugar, white flour, artificial sweeteners, and refined vegetable oils.

Sarcoidosis

This condition is officially listed as due to unknown causes. Yet, certainly, infection is the likely cause, and fungi and/or yeasts are the probable culprits. The fact is a careful assessment of the symptoms and manifestations of this disease clearly proves that infection is the primary factor. As would be expected from an infectious disease sarcoidosis attacks the entire body, however, the lungs are the main site of infestation.

The disease is regional, occurring mainly in the South, particularly in areas which have a humid climate, like the Carolinas, Georgia, Alabama, Mississippi, Kentucky, Virginia, and Florida. Incredibly, in Europe Sweden and Norway have the highest incidence. There is also a significant racial propensity. While the reason is unknown, people of African descent are ten times more likely to develop it than Caucasians.

The disease is manifested by sarcoids, which are lesions in the lungs, lymph nodes, and skin. There may be hundreds of these lesions in the lungs. These lesions induce inflammation and scarring. This is why cortisone and other immunosuppressive drugs, such as methotrexate, are frequently prescribed. Yet, under such treatment patients degenerate and usually die precipitously.

Sarcoidosis often is discovered due to the existence of skin lesions and/or swollen lymph glands. It may also be diagnosed upon routine X-ray, since it is often manifested by obvious spots on the lungs.

Treatment protocol

Fungal infection is the most likely cause of sarcoidosis. Currently, the type of fungus is unknown. The fact that fungus is the obvious cause becomes readily apparent by how and where it develops. Sarcoidosis occurs mainly in the Deep South, where humidity and mold counts are particularly high. The fungal cause is also revealed by the fact that it has a propensity to attack the lungs, the region of the body most vulnerable to fungal invasion. This is why antifungal spice extracts are the ideal treatment. Such extracts kill the entire range of molds, fungi, and yeasts. Plus, they exhibit significant anti-inflammatory properties. To reverse this condition take Oregacyn, two or more capsules twice daily. Natural anti-inflammatory agents are indicated. Take Bromazyme, a combination of papain and bromelain, 3 capsules twice daily on an empty stomach. Also, take crude natural bioflavonoids, such as Flavin-C, 3 or more capsules daily. The combination of enzymes plus bioflavonoids offers significant anti-inflammatory powers—without side effects. The typical treatments, that is cortisone, prednisone, and methotrexate, encourage the growth of fungi. Plus, these drugs are highly destructive to lung tissue. The fact is cortisone and prednisone dramatically encourage the growth of fungi. So does alcohol and refined sugar. If possible, strictly avoid their intake.

Scoliosis and Pott's disease: the hunch back syndromes

Neurologically, the lungs are one of the most sensitive of all organs. They are supplied by hundreds of miles of nerves. These nerves arise mainly from the spinal cord, although a few arise directly from the brain. Nerves control lung function. If they are irritated, the lungs also become irritated. Incredibly, this also happens in reverse: if the lungs are also irritated, they send messages through the nerves to the spine and ultimately the spinal muscles. This may lead to a condition known as spinal atrophy, which means that the spinal muscles degenerate.

Scoliosis and hunch back, that is kyphosis of the spine, are consequences of lung disease. The lungs lie directly behind the spine. If they are diseased, they send messages via the nervous system to it. These messages cause a kind of toxic stress, leading to destruction of the muscles, bones, and joints. Thus, in many instances a twisted and bowed back may not be primarily a spinal defect, that is the defect is evidence of diseases within the body, specifically the lungs. Thus, in order to cure the deformity or prevent it from worsening the lungs must be cleansed of all invaders as well as toxins.

The spine is one of the most important organs of the body. Normally, it is straight, that is it doesn't deviate from the midline. It has certain normal curvatures within this vertical structure. These are found in the neck, mid back, and lower lumbar regions. However, any degree of lateral, that is or side-ways, deviation is abnormal. This is known as scoliosis. This sideways curvature develops directly over the lung reflexes, that is the region of the spine supplied by the lungs' nerves. Scoliosis is pathological, and the likely origin for the pathology is the lung. Thus, disease in the lungs leads to disease of the spine.

Chronic infections of the lungs may be difficult to diagnose, and, thus, in an individual with scoliosis this may have never been considered as a cause. It is not the only cause. A severe deficiency of nutrients, particularly vitamin D and calcium, may result in scoliosis. Other minerals are needed for bone formation, particularly zinc and magnesium. Vitamin A is also required for the creation of healthy bone. Thus, individuals who are poorly nourished or who had poor nourishment in utero may develop this disorder. However, it is crucial to consider the infection connection. The infection may be hidden in the lungs, but it is also often disguised in the sinuses, tonsils, or adenoids or even the teeth.

Scoliosis may develop suddenly, usually after a severe infection. Other regions besides the lungs may be involved. Infections in the intestines, tonsils, ears, and adenoids have all been known to cause it. Tuberculosis is also a major factor. This may be a hidden cause, that is a low-grade type of tuberculosis that defies diagnosis. Yet, in a frail-appearing child, teenager, or young adult who develops scoliosis, the diagnosis of tuberculosis must be high on the list. This is especially true of the individual who is poorly nourished, of dark-skinned nature, and/or who fails to get sufficient sunshine.

Constipation has also been recognized as a cause. This may be due to the fact that toxins in the colon may be absorbed into the blood, poisoning lung tissue. The lung tissue acts as a sieve, absorbing toxins from the blood much like a living sponge. Cleansing of the colon may rapidly result in an improvement, even helping to induce a straightening of the spine. However, the cleansing program must be consistent, because if the toxic condition returns, the scoliosis worsens.

The germ that causes tuberculosis is a slow growing organism. Thus, it may be impossible to diagnose by cultures or blood tests. Plus, there are few if any reliable ways to discover its presence. Thus, symptoms and signs, that is obvious physical damage, can be relied upon to make the diagnosis. With the exception of that caused by obvious injury, a deformed or crooked spine in a youngster or young adult is a clear indication of chronic tuberculosis. There is not only deformity but also chronic pain. The most prominent symptom of undiagnosed spinal tuberculosis is pain. This pain may be felt in many areas. It could be a type of hip pain or possibly sciatica, that is pain down the back of the leg or hip. It could also be a type of chronic back pain. A vague type of abdominal pain that defies diagnosis may also represent it. Spinal stiffness, including ankylosing spondylitis, may be merely a representation of internal tubercular infection. Both the bones of the spinal column and the discs between the vertebrae are readily infected. However, even if the infection is in other regions, such as within the lungs or abdominal cavity, it may lead to scoliosis, spinal stiffness, or other spinal deformities. This is because tubercular infection causes massive scarring, which drags the vertebrae out of alignment. However, pain and deformity are only a few of the key symptoms of TB. Other common symptoms include in the early stages low body temperature in the morning, slight fever, especially in the afternoon, weight loss, slight persistent cough, and, later, persistent fever, chronic cough, coughing of blood or sputum, as well as, ultimately, increasing weight loss. Fistulas, that is openings in the skin which drain pus, are another important sign. Fulminant night sweats may also be an indicator. These may be so extreme as to soak the sheets.

Nutritional deficiency plays an enormous role in scoliosis. This is because deficiencies of amino acids, vitamins, minerals, and fatty acids greatly weaken immunity, increasing the risks for the development of chronic infection. Plus, the deficiencies cause a weakening of connective tissues. This weakening allows various germs to gain entry into the tissues, causing chronic infection. In tuberculosis and/or scoliosis dozens of nutrients are usually severely lacking. However, the primary deficiencies include a lack of amino acids, vitamin A, vitamin D, riboflavin, pantothenic acid, magnesium, zinc, and, particularly, vitamin C. The fact is a chronic lack of vitamin C greatly increases the risk for the development of both scoliosis and tuberculosis. Yet, the fat soluble vitamins are also severely lacking. Chronic depletion of vitamins A and D greatly increases the risks of TB infection. Few people realize that vitamins A and D are found in relatively few foods. The best sources are egg yolks, liver, kidney, fatty fish, sardines, herring, cod liver or its oil, and fatty milk products, all of which are rarely eaten today. Thus, significant deficiency is common.

In all cases of rigidity of the spine tuberculosis must be considered. Other infections may also be the cause, for instance, Lyme, staph, or candida. In this instance the normal curves of the spine disappear, a condition which may be described as "poker-back." This is due to inflammation in the joints. The inflammation results from infection. There are many sites for the infection, including the spinal column itself, the teeth, liver, spleen, adrenal glands, kidneys, lungs, intestines, sinuses, blood, and even the brain.

Treatment protocol

Tuberculosis, scoliosis, and spinal deformity require aggressive therapy. A prolonged period of supplementation, such as several months, may be necessary to reverse such disorders.

Massage and osteopathic treatments are of enormous benefit. The diet must be rich in highly nutritious foods. Only nutrient dense foods must be consumed. Follow the diet in *How to Eat Right and Live Longer*. The foods with the greatest nutrient density include eggs, whole milk products, cheese, red meat, poultry, fish, fresh fruit, and fresh vegetables. What's more, the intake of fresh whole organic milk is critical. The protein in milk greatly aids in boosting immunity. The exception is the individual who is allergic to it. In this instance the alternative is to consume fresh whole milk yogurt or perhaps goat's milk. Milk is also rich in riboflavin, which is needed for oxygen metabolism. Riboflavin aids in the prevention and reversal of TB: oxygen is toxic to this germ. If the riboflavin content of the lungs is high, so will be the oxygen utilization potential. Thus, a diet rich in riboflavin may act as a tuberculosis preventive. For more information in assessing your level of riboflavin and/or other vitamin deficiencies see the Web site, Nutritiontest.com. During the 1920s whole milk, rich in riboflavin, was an essential component for reversing TB.

A natural vegetable source of riboflavin in a concentrated form is available. Known as Wild Green Powerdrops, these drops are made exclusively from unprocessed wild greens. Therefore, they are completely different than the commercial greens and, thus, far more powerful. Plus, they contain wild nettle extract, invaluable for promoting healthy lungs. As a tonic and natural source of lung nourishing riboflavin, take 20 or more drops twice daily. This is the richest natural and/or vegetable source of this nutrient. This is a rare nutritional supplement: only a limited amount is available yearly, since it is picked totally from the wild by specially trained bushmen.

Milk is a mainstay in tuberculosis treatment. However, today, the milk is less nutritious than it was in the past. If fresh whole milk is available, it should be consumed on a daily basis. In sanatoriums fresh whole milk directly from cows or goats was fed to TB victims with tremendous results. For more information about the healing powers of fresh whole milk and other nutrient dense foods see the books, *Lifesaving Cures* and *How to Eat Right and Live Longer*.

Silicosis (silica deposits in the lungs)

This is perhaps the most frequent work-related disease of the lungs caused by industrial particles. Silica particles are highly toxic to lung tissue. Thus, they may cause severe scarring. When the lung tissues become scarred, they are weakened, and, as a result, these tissues become vulnerable to infection. In fact, tuberculosis is a common consequence of silicosis. So is chronic bronchitis. The fact is certain cases may present as the latter and, thus, be erroneously treated with antibiotics, cortisone, etc. What's more, occasionally silicosis may be misdiagnosed as asthma.

Silicosis is common in miners and also individuals who work in the sandblasting, concrete removal, demolition, and stone polishing industries. Thus, construction workers are its most frequent victims. While it was epidemic in such workers previously, today precautions have been taken which reduce the risks. Obviously, the greatest precaution is wearing protective masks. Silicosis may be one of the complications experienced by people in New York exposed to the Trade Center dust.

The symptoms of silicosis are rather vague and may mimic many other lung disorders, including bronchitis, emphysema, and asthma. It begins with shortness of breath, worsened by exertion. Wheezing and coughing usually follow, along with a weakening of the resistance against respiratory infections. As it worsens, sputum, which is grey colored or blood stained, may be produced. The final stage includes coughing of blood, which warns of tuberculosis. Chest X-rays may mimic the typical barrel chest of emphysema and, of course, reveal the characteristic silica nodules.

When the silica dust is inhaled, it is lodged in the deep recesses of the lungs. There, it is attacked by white blood cells, which attempt to remove it through the lymph. The white blood cells, as well as the lung's lymphatic glands, attempt to detoxify or destroy the silica. However, silica is a hard mineral and is difficult to decompose. Eventually, it plugs the lymphatics, leading to scarring. Thus, therapy must be aimed at stimulating the flow of lymph and preventing further scarring. What's more, efforts should be made to break down the scars through enzyme therapy as well as the inhalation of the appropriate essential oils.

If no treatment is given, the condition gradually worsens. Eventually, nodules filled with silica become visible on X-ray. The entire lung may eventually become fibrotic, and death usually occurs from infections, often tuberculous. This is where nature offers the most productive answers, since there is no medical cure for silicosis.

Essential oils, particularly spice oils, are an ideal therapy for this condition. Such oils act as solvents, denuding the silica molecules, essentially dissolving them. In other words, they cause the silica to be rendered water soluble. Spice oils offer the additional benefit of being antimicrobial. Italian research indicates that spice oils are actually able to dissolve silica deposits. Oils of wild oregano, rosemary, clove, cinnamon, juniper, and sage are all ideal for reversing this condition. Many of these oils are available in formulas, that is Respira Clenz and Oregacyn, which are multiple spice extracts.

Treatment protocol

Dust is the carrier for this disease, and that is where the danger lies. The simplest treatment is avoidance, that is taking precautions to avoid or minimize the inhalation of dust. This means wearing the appropriate masks at all times. Massive efforts must be made to help the body extract or dissolve the silica deposits. This may be a monumental task; however, it is not insurmountable. In order to dissolve scar tissue take Bromazyme, 2 or 3 capsules three times daily on an empty stomach. This contains a potent type of fruit enzyme capable of dissolving scar tissue. Also, take vitamin E, 400 I. U. daily. Essential oils have solvent properties, and, thus, they help dissolve organic compounds, including silica deposits. Oils of oregano, rosemary, sage, cloves, and juniper all exhibit these properties. Take P73 oil of wild oregano (the Maximum Strength variety is the best), five to ten drops twice daily. Also, take a special combination of these oils, Respira Clenz, 20 drops twice daily. This is highly respected by doctors as an effective agent for lung support. For additional power take the multiple spice extract, that is Oregacyn, two capsules twice daily. Crude wild greens also assist lung function. Take the Wild Green powerdrops, 20 drops twice daily. The latter is high in natural riboflavin, which is needed for oxygen transport in the lungs. The wild greens is a rare nutritional supplement and is not available in stores. To order call 1-800-243-5242 or in Canada (Bulk Food Warehouse) 1-905-634-9480.

Sinusitis

This is one of modern humankind's greatest epidemics. Sinusitis afflicts tens of millions of North Americans. It is usually a chronic ailment, seemingly unresponsive to any type of medication. It may be defined as inflammation and/or swelling in the sinuses. These toxic effects are usually caused by infection.

The sinuses, along with the nasal passages, are a key organ of respiration. Both the nose and the sinuses act as radiators, warming the air. They also act as filters, removing particles that could severely damage the lungs. As a sort of air conditioner they add moisture to the air, as necessary, since air which is too dry may also damage the lungs. The nasal and sinus membranes produce mucus, which is a key secretion for protecting the lungs from toxicity. This mucus helps trap harmful particles, as well as germs, so they may be detoxified and/or destroyed. Thus, in essence the nose and sinuses are a sort of house cleaner for the lungs, keeping these organs from being burdened by harmful agents.

The cilia are a fascinating organ system found within the nasal and sinus regions. These are delicate hair-like organs, but they are not stiff or coarse. They are like tiny velvet fibers. Their job is to cleanse the mucus, acting essentially like a living conveyor belt. They constantly mobilize inhaled "garbage" towards the stomach, to prevent it from entering the lungs.

There are several sinus cavities. Some are located just above the eyes on the lower forehead. Others are located just under the cheekbone. Still, others are located on either side of the nose and behind the nose deep in the facial bones.

Sinus disorders may exhibit a wide range of symptoms. The symptoms are so diverse and/or bizarre that the proper diagnosis is frequently missed. Headache is perhaps the most common symptom, along with pressure in the face or forehead. Stuffiness of the nose is also a signal. Post nasal drip may indicate the existence of chronic sinus infection and/or allergy. Also, there is often the complaint of thick mucus at the back of the throat that simply cannot be cleared. Facial pain may have its primary origin in sinus infection as well as pain in the teeth. Common patterns of pain include pain over one eye, generalized head pain, one-sided headache, pain on the tip of the head, pain in the ear, neck pain, pain between the shoulder blades, and arm pain. Infection or inflammation in the sphenoid sinus, which is located behind the nose fairly close to the inner ear, may create symptoms in the ear. Dr. Albert Seltzer, sinus specialist, describes a case of a woman who complained of noises in her ear, sounding like a foghorn or at other times like a whistle. Treating the sinus disorder cured the symptoms. Even colds may have their origin in sinus problems, especially in the person who suffers from repeated bouts. Dr. Seltzer describes another odd case: a person complaining of dark spots before the eyes. When the sinus infection was cured, the eye problems disappeared. It is easy to comprehend from the diversity of symptoms why the diagnosis is often elusive.

Traditionally, bacterial infections have been regarded as the primary cause of sinusitis. Yet, antibiotics have been found to be largely ineffective. This is because the model for the treatment of sinus disorders has been erroneous. This was recently proved at the Mayo Clinic. Doctors at the Clinic were stymied as to why sinus patients failed to improve despite intensive antibiotic therapy. They cultured the sinuses and failed to find bacteria. Instead, they found molds. In fact, 40 different molds and yeasts were recovered. The molds instigated pain, irritation, and inflammation. The conclusion of these investigators was that chronic sinus disease is due to fungal infection. Antibiotics are useless against fungi, in fact, these drugs enhance fungal growth.

Dental disorders may lead to sinus infections. The upper teeth are directly connected to the roof of the sinuses. If the teeth are infected, the toxins and germs readily enter the sinuses, causing a wide range of symptoms. Some of the more prominent symptoms include stuffy sinuses, sinus drainage, sinus headaches, facial pain, pain around the eye, and even seemingly remote symptoms, like arm, hip, leg, and back pain. Dr. Seltzer describes numerous cases where when the dental problems were cured, the sinus problems completely disappeared.

Sinus disorders may arise after flying. This is caused by the tremendous forces resulting from pressure changes in the ears, most prominently occurring during takeoff and landing. The eustachian tube between the nose and ears attempts to equalize the pressure so that it won't damage the head, that is the brain. The pressure changes that occur within this tube lead to swelling, or they may force nasal or sinus secretions deeper into the sinuses or even into the inner ear. If secretions enter the inner ear, infection may develop. In adults this infection has been known to cause hearing loss: even deafness.

Treatment protocol

Oregacyn is a potent therapy for sinusitis. It helps halt excessive secretions while destroying noxious microbes. To correct this problem take one to two capsules twice daily. For difficult conditions take more, like 3 or 4 capsules three times daily. This dosage is acceptable for 2 weeks, then reduce it to 1 to 4 capsules daily. Also, take oil of wild oregano, five or more drops twice daily. For difficult conditions increase the dosage. The oil may also be rubbed on the sinus regions, like the forehead or under the cheek bones. Or, it may also be inhaled directly. Extremely difficult conditions may require the use of the Maximum Strength oil of wild oregano. Take ten or more drops twice daily under the tongue. After placing it under the tongue, hold it against the tissues with the tip of the tongue for at least a minute. This will aid in penetration, because under the tongue administration gets the oil directly into the blood. Also, saturate a Q-Tip with the oil, and gently place in the nose for a few moments. This direct treatment may rapidly eliminate sinus symptoms and even help reverse the disease. If flying, be sure to take an Oregacyn just before take-off and another capsule just before landing. Use the Germ-a-Clenz to spray down any suspect item or region. Pump-spray it high into the air in any contaminated room.

Smallpox

This disease is caused by a virus known medically as the variola virus. This virus is the largest known to infect humans. While it is large compared to other viruses, it is still tiny by cellular standards. Some three million smallpox viruses fit on the tip of a pen.

From pictures it would appear that smallpox is a skin disease. This is misleading, because, while there are obvious skin lesions, it has a viscous effect upon the entire body, including the internal organs.

Historically, smallpox was perhaps the most feared, as well as common, of all communicable diseases. It is the greatest infectious killer of all time. In fact, it is such an aggressive killer that it altered the course of the Roman Empire, accelerating its decline. It also changed the course of history in America. The Native Americans, who had no immunity to it, were largely destroyed by this disease. Incredibly, they were precisely victims of biological warfare. Europeans, notably the Englishman Sir Jeffrey Amhurst, deliberately introduced the virus into native communities. They did so by sending the natives the "gift" of smallpox-infested blankets, that is blankets used by smallpox victims. These blankets were infested with insects, which transmitted the disease. As a result, millions of natives died, which made the conquering of their race far easier. The Europeans had sufficient history of exposure and, therefore, immunity, while the natives, a virgin population, were devoid of it. In some regions 90% of the native population was destroyed. The natives were an impediment to the settlement objectives of the early colonists. Thus, this biological warfare led to what was essentially a culling of the native population and, thus, the rapid expansion of Western civilization.

Smallpox is a frightening disease, largely because of what it does cosmetically to the body. It may cause permanent scarring, especially on the face and torso. It is also feared, because of the intense pain and misery it causes. When it strikes, people become totally bedridden. Plus, they experience severe pain and a bizarre burning sensation on the skin and mucus membranes.

Smallpox is currently extinct in the United States and other Western countries. In fact, it has apparently been eradicated globally. However, stores of smallpox germs exist in microbiological labs, where they are held for research or as potential biological agents. Thus, if a deliberate attempt were made to seed this virus, a localized or even global epidemic could occur.

When smallpox strikes, it is particularly dangerous for children as well as the fetus. Here, it is highly fatal. However, with adults the fatality rate is also high: some 30%. Blacks are unusually susceptible, as are Native Americans. However, currently, virtually all people globally, especially Westerners, are highly vulnerable. This is particularly true of individuals with weakened immunity or who are taking immunocompromising drugs such as Cortisone or chemotherapeutic drugs.

The germ gains entrance into the body through the lungs: Thus, sneezing, breathing, and coughing primarily disseminate it. Merely talking could transmit it. However, there are few obvious lung signs. Rather, the obvious signs are in the skin and mucous membranes. Pustules occur on the skin, and ulcers appear on the mucous membranes. The skin may suffer tiny hemorrhages. The skin lesions may become boil-like, and they may coalesce into large boil-like patches. The lungs usually only become symptomatic as the result of secondary bacterial infections. As the infection extends the internal organs may swell and hemorrhage. If the internal swelling and hemorrhaging becomes extreme, death may rapidly ensue. In summary the signs and symptoms of smallpox include in order of occurrence:

- sudden sickness manifested by weakness and fever
- sickness to the stomach, vomiting, diarrhea, pain all over, headaches, and (in children) convulsions
- spiking of the fever, restlessness, sleeplessness, and delirium
- eruption of a rash, first on the face and forearms
- eruption on the upper arms and trunk, followed by the spread to the buttocks and legs
- formation of red vesicles, which become hard
- the vesicles ultimately become full of pus-like fluid, then burst, after which they become encrusted

Smallpox can enter the body insidiously. In other words, the existence of infection may not be readily evident. This is because smallpox has a relatively long incubation period: about

15 days. When it does initiate, it may begin with chills, utter exhaustion, prostration (can't get out of bed), skin boils and pustules, which tend to grow bigger and eventually touch each other, severe pain, and fever. The fever rapidly rises and then gradually falls. It can be extreme: up to 107 degrees. As it falls the skin eruptions occur. These eruptions begin as pimples, then boils, then pus pimples (pustules), and then encrusted lesions. As described by T. J. Ritter, M. D., in *Mother's Remedies*, published in 1910, any non-vaccinnated person who is directly exposed will contract this dreaded disease.

However, mass vaccinations are not without risk. The sudden and unbridled imposition of vaccinations in the entire populace could lead to a wide range of ill effects: even thousands of deaths. The authorities who promote such mass vaccinations rarely if ever popularize the degree of untoward effects. This is because the attitude taken regarding mass vaccinations is that what is supposedly good for humanity at large is worth any risk, that is the risk for side effects and loss of life. However, this is merely advertising jargon. No evidence is provided of a scientifically proven benefit. What's more, the production of vaccinations is an enormous business. Thus, vested interests promote vaccinations for financial gain. In fact, billions stand to be made, literally overnight, if national vaccination programs are ordained. Even so, it is true that direct exposure is the most risky type. Thus, because the smallpox vesicles are highly infective, special precautions must be taken in order to prevent the spread of this disease. Direct exposure to these vesicles is a major means for transmission. Here is where essential oils are of critical value. They offer significant antiseptic actions, sterilizing the air. On the skin they offer potent sterilization. When taken internally, they also sterilize tissues and internal organs, including the blood. They are particularly valuable as antiseptic rubs. They may also be sprayed into the air as emulsified aerosols such as Germ-a-Clenz.

There is no certain evidence that vaccinations cure or prevent the disease. In the Western world the incidence declines in concert with improvements in sanitation, that is improved housing, reduction of poverty, chlorination of water, proper disposal of garbage, improved food supply, etc. According to J. H. Greer, M.D., author of *A Physician in the House*, in the United States smallpox was known as a "filth disease", one propagated by unsanitary conditions. The fact is it was largely a disease of the poor and lower class, and it was routinely fatal in the impoverished and/or malnourished, that is where there was poor attention to proper cleanliness, nutrition, and hygiene. Of note, the regular intake in such poorly nourished people of vitamin C-rich foods, such as fresh fruits and vegetables, was exceptionally low. As a result, the regular intake of vitamin C was compromised. This lack of vitamin C greatly compromised immunity, increasing the risks for smallpox infection.

Thus, in the current global climate smallpox is likely to make a comeback, since there has been a vast dilemma of global strife, war, and poverty, as well as the war-induced destruction of infrastructure, sanitation, etc. The fact is this is the ideal climate for the regeneration of this disease. What's more, apparently, outbreaks are being reported in the war-torn regions of the former Yugoslavia. Afghanistan, replete with sanitation-poor refugee camps, is yet another likely climate for it.

Dr. Greer continues that proper sanitation was only a 20th century science. He provides compelling proof that sanitation improvements were the primary reasons for the elimination of smallpox as well as cholera and typhoid fever. For instance, he notes, no one would ever consider that vaccinations cured cholera. Yet, this scourge, which previously struck every few years, killing thousands, is now virtually extinct, without vaccinations. He continues that there is always some opportunist who only wishes he would have made up and administered a vaccine simultaneous to cholera's or some other communicable disease's elimination. Then, he would have taken credit for "stamping out" this disease, thereby creating a future source of revenue for the medical profession. Based upon Dr. Greer's vast experience he makes a rather profound statement, that is that "vaccination does not give the least protection against smallpox, but on the contrary it increases the liability."

Dr. L. M. Bush, writing in *Common Sense Health*, is also against routine vaccination. As early as the 1930s he observed highly toxic reactions to such vaccines, causing him to seriously question their validity. In his chapter entitled Serums and Vaccines he claims, "The practice of medicine has always been subject to various fads and fancies...few methods of treatment have survived for many years. If patients today were given many of the forms of treatment advocated thirty years ago, it would be considered very unscientific and...years from now some of the things we do today will be considered equally bad." One of those very things, according to Dr. Bush, is commercial vaccines. Furthermore, he claims sanitation and hygiene are fully responsible for the rapid decline of smallpox, not vaccinations. Ominously, he titles one of his sections, "...Relation to Increase of Cancer." Here, he carefully surmises how the sudden rise in the United States of cancer is directly tied to commercial vaccines. The rise in cancer noted in the early part of the century, that is from the 1920s to the 1950s, coincides directly with the injection in Americans of a wide range of serums and vaccines. These potions, he notes, are derived from animal blood and secretions. Thus, they, are notoriously contaminated. Such contamination introduces microbial proteins, genetic material, and various unknown germs, which may invade human cells. There, they overcome the cellular machinery, causing irritation and inflammation. They also readily attack the genetic material. Such irritation, says Dr. Bush, ultimately leads to cancer. Furthermore, he asks a curious question: why are soldiers, who are supposed to be the healthiest specimens of Western civilization, often the sickest? Why do such individuals frequently develop chronic disease as well as cancer? Dr. Bush directly attributes it to the fact that they were the primary recipients of commercial vaccines.

Today, there is yet another compelling question. Why are those who tout vaccines bandying about the concept of the individual's need to be vaccinated in order to be "responsible?" It is as if a person is to feel guilty for refusing vaccinations. These supposed experts claim that if you fail to get vaccinated, you could put others directly at risk. They claim it is a "patriotic" duty to be vaccinated. However, how could a person who refused the vaccination be a risk, especially to those who are vaccinated, that is if vaccination truly works? In fact, it is likely to be the contrary, that is the vaccinated individual could shed the injected germs upon the healthier un-vaccinated individual. What's more, those who are vaccinated will suffer ill health and, thus, be a burden on civilization, while the un-vaccinated person will be stronger and, therefore, more productive.

This is perhaps why the powers of home remedies and natural cures are rarely discussed in government circles. The federal government is under extreme financial distress. Thus, it is beholden to the financial concerns of those in power and readily bows to the interests of the few. Public interest is rarely if ever the motive. While it is possible that the World Health Organization may have initially saved lives through its vaccination program, the chronic ill effects of its program are dire. Perhaps the rapid death rate in Africa, where hundreds of thousands die daily from AIDS and other viral syndromes, is due to the previous and current mass vaccinations of a population, which was unable to tolerate the introduction of such a vast amount of microbially-contaminated injections. Future research is needed to document the role of vaccinations in the astronomically high death rate in Africa. However, in the future the safety of vaccines should be carefully assessed before they are administered.

There is a science to protecting the body from ill effects of vaccinations. This is the science of immune protection and immune stimulation. In other words, the immune system can be greatly strengthened, and this can be an effective defense. Immune strengthening fails to interfere with the potential utility of vaccinations. It only helps prevent toxic effects. As a result of the vaccination, an immunity is developed, and the immune system recognizes the germs in case they attempt to invade the body in the future. However, the immune stimulation resulting from the vaccination stresses the body, and this can deplete its powers. Thus, vitamins which bolster immunity, such as vitamin C, vitamin B-6, pantothenic acid, and vitamin A, help replenish the depletion, while protecting the body from the toxic effects of vaccinations. What's more, such vitamins, if well supplied in the cells, may prevent the occurrence of small-pox and similar diseases. This again illustrates the flaw of relying upon mass vaccination exclusively. Nutritional education and, thus, the regular intake of the appropriate nutrients greatly "immunizes" the body from communicable diseases. The regular intake of the aforementioned vitamins, as well as the appropriate vitamin-rich foods, could prevent the need for mass vaccination. Yet, at a minimum if you are forced to undergo a new vaccine, especially if you are an individual, you must take immune bolstering nutrients. The most important of these are vitamin C, vitamin A, pyridoxine, pantothenic acid, and selenium. Yet, the most powerful immunization is the use of natural substances with germ-destructive power.

Certain herbal medicines help reverse vaccine toxicity. Wild oregano is the most powerful of these. As a protection take a few drops of oil of wild Oreganol under the tongue after any vaccination. In addition, rub the oil on the injection site once or twice daily. Make a pack for the site with the oil plus raw honey. Cover with a Telfa pad and change every 24 hours. Also, take Oregacyn, 2 or 3 capsules twice daily. This is known as the "cleansing herb" of the ancient law, that is of the Old Testament. Thus, as demonstrated by the divine source it can be relied upon to purge or detoxify unwanted residues.

Before synthetic drugs became established dietary and herbal therapies were relied upon in the treatment and prevention of smallpox. It was discovered that adding fresh milk to the diet resulted in a rapid improvement. This is probably because milk is rich in key vitamins, like riboflavin, vitamin A, and vitamin D, which are difficult to procure in other foods. It is also an excellent source of amino acids, so direly needed for immune health. Spearmint and peppermint teas were used for gastric or abdominal symptoms. Honey with sage tea was used as a gargle for irritated mouth or throat. Peruvian bark was administered for severe exhaustion. A tea made from the old southern remedy, sassafras bark plus catnip, was used to accelerate the eruptions so they would heal more quickly. According to Gunn's *Family Physician and Home Book of Health* black cohosh, also known as native rattle root, was "an important remedy in smallpox." The patient was given it regularly from the time of the first eruption until healing began. According to the editors it keeps the eruption from invading the deep tissues and causes it to be purged out of the skin. A native root compound is now available. Called Spirit Drops it is a potent root extract for regenerating and healing the body. Useful for a wide range of conditions, it would be an invaluable aid in the reversal and/or prevention of smallpox. While wild oregano is the mainstay as the natural treatment, the Spirit Drops is an ideal adjunct. These drops are highly aromatic, plus they are soothing. This makes this tonic an ideal therapy for sick children. This is a rare herbal supplement, unavailable in stores. To order call 1-800-243-5242.

According to *Vitalogy,* a book written in 1930 by E. H. Ruddin, M.D., the Paris Academy of Medicine described an herbal tonic that was nearly always curative. The main ingredient was the herb foxglove, the same one from which digitalis is made. Tartaric acid, the main acidic compound in grapes and grape extracts, was regarded by English nurses as a significant cure. This may be found naturally in crude red grape extracts such as Resvitanol. The fact is Resvitanol is the top natural source of tartaric acid. Red grape juice is also a good source, but it is weak compared to Resvitanol as an immune stimulant. American nurses used a different acid, vinegar water, to soothe facial and head lesions. Smallpox was known to infect the eyes, causing blindness. Dr. Ruddin describes the frequent use of rose water essence to prevent eye infection/damage.

Currently, individuals throughout the Western world are receiving smallpox vaccines. This is the first time in decades that such vaccines have been administered. Incredibly, the vaccine fails to contain the true smallpox virus. Instead, it contains a relative, known as vaccinia. This is one of many viruses from the so-called Poxvirus family. According to L. E. Hanson, Ph.D., in his book, *Diseases Transmitted from Animals to Man*, Pox viral infections have been known in humans and animals for centuries. He indicates that the true reservoir for these viruses are animals, notably monkeys, pigs, horses, and cattle. The Pox viruses from these animals can readily infect humans. These viruses are highly contagious and, once introduced to a host, can readily infect other individuals. Their biological nature and structure is complex and largely unknown. Once they invade the body their mechanism of action is also unknown.

Specifically, the current smallpox vaccine is made using the animal virus, vaccinia. Hanson notes that this is a genetically modified animal virus, in other words, it is a type of man-made agent. What's more, it contains several unknown viruses. According to the Journal of the American Medical Association the smallpox vaccine is contaminated with numerous other animal viruses.

Treatment protocol

If smallpox or vaccinia strikes, take the P73 oil of wild oregano aggressively. Take it under the tongue, a few drops every hour or even every half hour. If respiratory symptoms develop, take Oregacyn, two or more capsules several times daily. Use the oil topically on any region. Eat large quantities of onions and garlic, as the sulfur in them helps kill germs, plus it speeds the healing of skin. For generalized immune support take organic selenium, 600 mcg daily, vitamin A, 10,000 I.U. daily, and vitamin C, 1000 mg twice daily. Also, take a crude natural vitamin C/flavonoid supplement, since crude natural vitamin C speeds the healing of tissues and is retained superiorly in the body, for instance, Flavin-C, three capsules every two hours. To eradicate the prostration and weakness take Royal Kick (premium-grade royal jelly), three capsules every few hours. Get a diffuser and add essential oils, like oils of lavender, neroli, rosemary, oregano, sage, etc., and disseminate throughout the air. Also, spray Germ-a-Clenz throughout the house. Spray it on furnace or air conditioning filters. Pump-spray it about the bedroom at bedtime. This spray is exceptionally effective in halting the spread of this germ.

While the likelihood of a natural outbreak of smallpox is minimal, now, as a result of the vaccination program, populations may suffer the disease. This is where the wild oregano can prove invaluable, because it destroys both smallpox and the vaccinia virus, that is the type used in the vaccination. To reiterate the mainstay of treatment is the Oregacyn and oregano oil: all other supplements are secondary. For topical treatment of pustules or other wounds use wild raw honey. Mix a few drops of oregano oil (or Spirit Drops) in the honey, and apply to any lesion. The healing will be dramatic. Plus, the honey-oregano applications will prevent scar tissue formation, whether on pustules or the vaccination site. What's more, Oregacyn and/or oregano oil are ideal as antidotes to the vaccine. Thus, the minimum basic protocol is:

Internally: Oregacyn, one or more capsules three or more times daily. Oreganol oil, ten or more drops under the tongue three or more times daily.

Topically: Oreganol oil or cream rubbed on lesions twice daily. Or, a combination of the oil plus raw honey applied to any lesion or injection site. Dressings may be changed daily or twice daily.

Do not be concerned about the consequences or toxicity of smallpox. Do not fret over the issue of disfigurement. All can be prevented by the timely use of wild oregano extracts. Topically, crude raw honey completely prevents scar formation.

Smoke inhalation

This fire-related disaster happens to thousands of North Americans daily. High levels of smoke poison the lungs, causing severe tissue damage. However, the damage caused by cigarettes is far more common and significant than disaster-related smoke damage.

Cigarette smoke causes significant tissue damage. Secondhand smoke is nearly as dangerous as actual smoking. Toxic hydrocarbons enter the lungs, causing inflammation and irritation. These hydrocarbons are among the most potent carcinogens known. One of these, nitrosamine, is so toxic that the amount of this chemical that would fit on the tip of a pin is enough to induce cancer. Yet, there are thousands of chemicals in smoke, including nitrosamines, and all of them are toxic.

Smoke can rapidly damage the lungs. However, with the use of natural medicines much of the damage can be reversed. The lungs are in dire need of antioxidants in order to cleanse themselves of toxins. Otherwise, the toxins accumulate, poisoning the lung cells. The natural antioxidants, vitamins, minerals, enzymes, and spice extracts act as biological cleansing agents, empowering the white blood cells and other cellular aid workers in their efforts to remove accumulated poisons. The intake of these antioxidants and edible spice oils makes an enormous impact on the rate of healing of lung tissue. The edible spice oils are so effective that they can be used in the midst of a crisis to prevent severe disease and/or fatality. The most potent of these is a special type of antioxidant oregano called Oreganol Antioxidant Blend. This provides enormous cellular protection. It is a cellular antioxidant formula specifically for preventing and reversing cellular damage. According to research at the USDA the components of Oreganol Antioxidant Blend offer the most potent cellular antioxidant protection known. Oreganol Antioxidant Blend is made through a special process, which concentrates the antioxidant fractions of certain spicy herbs, notably wild oregano and rosemary. ORAC testing, the standard in the industry, proves that the antioxidant form of Oreganol is the most potent antioxidant formula ever tested. It scored nearly 3000 points, some three times greater than any other substance previously tested. Well known natural antioxidant foods, such as pomegranates, blueberries, and strawberries, were insignificant in comparison. The fact is as an antioxidant Oreganol is incomparably more powerful than any vitamin or mineral, including vitamin E, selenium, and beta carotene.

Treatment protocol

To reverse the toxicity of acute exposure take Oreganol Antioxidant Blend, one or more dropperfuls twice daily. Also, take Oregacyn, 2 or more capsules as needed. For an acute crisis take a capsule or 2 as often as every hour and also take the Oreganol Antioxidant Blend more frequently. During an acute attack use it more aggressively, like every few minutes. Take also 10 or more drops of edible oil of rosemary in an olive oil base two times daily or as needed. While vitamins A, C, E, and beta carotene are crucial for smoke detoxification, spice extracts are far more powerful. The Oregacyn and Oreganol Antioxidant Blend are aggressive for reversing smoke-induced lung damage. Also, the mineral selenium is an aggressive smoke antagonist: take 400 to 600 mcg of organically bound selenium daily. For acute smoke toxicity take a higher amount, for instance, 400 mcg two or three times daily. High doses of selenium can only be taken for a short period, like a few weeks. A safe daily dose is 200 to 400 mcg.

Tonsillitis

The tonsils are one of the most critical immunological organs, perhaps the most critical of all. They are the guardians to the gate of entry: the oral, digestive, and respiratory cavities. Their role is to help the body capture toxic invaders, especially germs.

It is a travesty that the usefulness of these glands has been disregarded. The tonsils were made for a specific purpose. They are the body's immunological sentinels, protecting the gate of entry from noxious invaders. Yet, for decades physicians regarded them to be of no significance and, thus, frequently prescribed their removal. However, now it is known that the tonsils serve a critical function and that they should only be removed as a last resort. In fact, every effort must be made to retain them and, thus, to cure tonsular illnesses with non-surgical therapies.

For decades both doctors and patients regarded the tonsils as useless. In fact, they regarded them as disease-breeding. A surgical crusade was begun in the 1950s to remove them. During the height of this folly in the United States and Canada as many as 2.5 million people per year, mostly children, had their tonsils surgically removed. The crusade was largely financially motivated. Yet, the *Journal of the American Medical Association,* the most orthodox of all medical journals, claims that "Tonsils...are protective organs and should not be removed."

The tonsils are simply a mass of lymph tissue. However, their function is vital. They are rather large in childhood, when they are needed the most, and gradually shrink with age. In the elderly they are tiny but are often still functional. They should not be removed with the exception of life threatening illnesses.

The tonsils have an excellent blood supply, needed to deliver white blood cells and extract toxins. Naturally, as a result of their function they may become inflamed and swollen. Yet, this is far from a cause for alarm. In other words children do not die from swollen tonsils. They are just performing their role of cleansing and detoxifying poisons and microbes. This swelling and pain are also a normal consequence and, other than the discomfort, are no cause for alarm. These glands do the job for which they were created: trapping and draining off infection and helping to prepare the immune system for future assaults.

The tonsils are the human body's most important sentries, guarding the gate to the vulnerable internal organs. Their removal greatly impairs immunity and increases the risks for chronic and serious diseases, particularly fungal infections, chronic bacterial infections, intestinal disorders, and even cancer. To decrease the swelling there is an effective technique. Make an oregano oil-salt water gargle. Take 5 drops of Oreganol in a 6 to 8 oz glass of salt water. Gargle repeatedly.

Swollen or sore tonsils act as a warning of infection elsewhere in the body, for instance, the teeth, sinuses, digestive tract, or lungs. They are a miraculous organ, because of their ability to warn of potential problems as well as help prevent future illnesses. One article reports that if infected teeth or sinuses are cured, tonsillar function returns to normal. Thus, removing the tonsils fails to treat the cause: chronic infection hidden somewhere else in the body.

Modern medicine has basically failed to correctly treat individuals with tonsil and adenoid infections. Millions of tonsils are removed merely on the supposition that colds and sore throats would be lessened. A study of nearly 4500 children proved that removal of tonsils failed to reduce the incidence of any type of respiratory disease, including colds, ear infections, and bronchitis. What's more, their removal increases the likelihood for the development of chronic diseases, particularly allergic illnesses, sinus disorders, asthma, attention deficit disorder, and autism. Their removal also increases the risk for development of diseases in adulthood, including immune deficiency, arthritis, and cancer. The fact has been documented in scientific studies that there is a slight increase above normal in such diseases in those whose tonsils are removed.

Treatment protocol

The tonsils are readily cleansed through the intake of potent natural antiseptics. Take oil of wild Oreganol, five to ten drops twice daily under the tongue. For severe cases take the oil several times daily, like five drops every hour or two. Use an oreganol-salt water gargle several times daily. The Oregacyn is extremely aggressive and may be needed to help shrink the tonsillar swelling and eradicate deep-seated infections.

If infected teeth are suspected as a source for the infection, rub P73 oil of wild oregano on the involved region(s) once or twice daily. Add a drop or two of the oil to a toothbrush and brush gently. For sinus disorders take Oregacyn, one or two capsules twice daily. Continue this amount for at least two months. Also, take oil of wild oregano, 3 to 5 drops under the tongue twice daily. For tough situations take it more frequently, five or six times daily.

Tuberculosis

This is one of the most devastating of all diseases. Incredibly, it afflicts as much as one third of the human race. In the United States it is gradually increasing in incidence, soon to rival its previous prominence—soon to again become a devastating epidemic.

The disease is caused by a germ known medically as *Mycobacterium tuberculosis*, apparently a type of bacteria. There is some doubt about this, however, as this bizarre, destructive, slow growing germ somewhat resembles a fungus. The name reveals this: Myco (fungal) bacterium. According to the editors of the *Introduction to Respiratory Diseases*, National

Tuberculosis and Respiratory Disease Association, the tuberculosis germ may be regarded as sort of a fungus-bacteria. This may explain the insidious nature of this infection. It also explains the relative resistance of the germ to standard antibiotic therapy. In the earlier 1900s when millions of Americans were afflicted tuberculosis was known as consumption, because it literally consumed the individual, gradually destroying the vital tissues. Most people regard tuberculosis as only a lung disease but, in fact, it greatly and negatively affects the entire body. With time the disease causes the decay of all of the organs, even the bones, leaving the individual weakened, debilitated, and exhausted. Ultimately, it kills the individual.

The bacteria which causes tuberculosis, Mycobacterium tuberculosis, is descended from similar germs which have infested cattle for eons. Ultimately, the germ mutated, adapting to human tissue. Once adapted, it has developed the capacity to permanently infect human populations.

The infective powers of TB are largely a consequence of its physical structure. This germ is surrounded with a kind of biological rind, making it highly resistant to the immune system. In other words, its coating prevents the immune system from readily attacking it. The white cells essentially slip off of its greasy coat.

Tuberculosis has made a rather massive comeback. In the United States it is endemic in certain hospitals, especially those with large populations of AIDS patients. Even relatively healthy individuals are developing it. Vegetarians are at a high risk, because a lack of high grade protein diminishes immunity. Plus, complete avoidance of animal foods causes stomach atrophy. Such damage to the stomach halts the production of stomach acid, needed to sterilize food. Thus, if tubercular germs are ingested, they gain entrance to the blood and/or organs, causing infection.

Tuberculosis is readily spread on airlines. The air filters in the jets/planes may become contaminated. If air is stagnant or if filters spew the germs, virtually anyone on the plane may become infected. This is perhaps the most common mode of inoculation. It may manifest as little more than an insidious cough and fatigue. Hundreds, rather, thousands, of flight attendants have become infected in this manner, and most of them have yet to be diagnosed. This is because it may take several years for the symptoms of tuberculosis to manifest.

The tuberculosis germ readily hides. Its main site may not be the lungs: it may be the teeth or sinuses, even the kidneys. Thus, excellent oral hygiene as well as proper health of the sinuses, perhaps through regular sinus gavage, may be necessary to eradicate and/or prevent this illness.

The symptoms of TB are often difficult to recognize. It is often a cause of hidden infection or disease. Plus, while it usually primarily afflicts the lungs, it may cause disease in virtually any organ. Signs and symptoms of TB which are only rarely recognized include spinal stiffness, stiffness of the joints, knee or hip pain on one side, chronic sinus problems, night sweats, a draining fistula, muscle wasting, exhaustion, poor posture, scoliosis, and poor appetite. When severe it may also cause deformities of the spinal column and neck, including scoliosis.

Treatment protocol

Tuberculosis is one of the most difficult of all illnesses to cure. It is chronic which means that it is a slow growing, smoldering infection, which is difficult to eradicate. The unassisted immune system often fails to cure it. However, antiseptic spice extracts offer hope for a cure.

The key is to take the supplements regularly; never miss a dose. This is essential, because it is critical to maintain proper blood levels of the antiseptic to eradicate this infection. This is a chronic and significant disease, and it must be taken seriously. It requires a monumental effort to cure, and consistency is the key. As the most powerful natural antiseptic available, take Oregacyn, 2 capsules three times daily. For tougher cases massive doses may be required, for instance, 3 capsules four times daily. Such large doses of Oregacyn must be taken with meals. Take also Super Strength oil of wild oregano, 20 drops under the tongue two or three times daily. For difficult cases take larger amounts, such as 20 to 40 drops three or four times daily. Get as much sunlight as possible. If you must spend much of your time indoors, buy full spectrum lights, and install them in all fixtures/lamps. Keep windows open as much as possible. Eat large amounts of high protein food. If you can tolerate it, drink a quart of whole organic milk daily. If milk is poorly tolerated, eat yogurt, four cups daily. Follow the diet in Dr. Cass Ingram's *How to Eat Right and Live Longer*. Take a natural vitamin C supplement, such as Flavin-C, about 200 mg of natural vitamin C daily (follow the label claims on the bottles to know the amount to take). As a potent cleansing tonic take the Wild Green Powerdrops, 4 droppers daily. This also provides natural riboflavin, needed by the lungs for regeneration.

For excellent sinus health do a daily sinus gavage. Snort

saline water into the nostrils two or three times daily. Press one nostril closed, and inhale the saline water with the other; allow the fluid to either come out through the mouth or back through the nostrils. Also, oil of wild oregano and oil of wild bay leaf are excellent for sinus cleansing. Place a drop or two in the salt water. Or, take a few drops under the tongue twice daily.

Multiple spice extracts offer the greatest hope for a cure. Drugs are largely impotent, plus they exhibit numerous side effects. Blindness is a common side effect of anti-tuberculosis drugs. Spice extracts have been shown to kill TB germs. The fact is they are capable of sterilizing sewage. These heat-producing extracts are among the most powerful germ killing substances known, and, since they are from edible plants, they are far safer than other medicinal herbs and certainly infinitely safer than drugs. As immune-boosting tonics these extracts are extremely beneficial for TB patients. As a result of their regular use, usually, energy, strength, and lung function improve within days.

Today, with standard therapy TB is nearly impossible to cure. This is largely due to the emergence of drug-resistant forms. It is the wild-source spice extracts, which offer the only hope for a cure. Recent experiments at Georgetown University indicate that germs of the tubercular family routinely succumb to these extracts. Ideal results are seen with a variety of spices. Such multiple spice extracts offer the best potency against drug resistant forms of TB. Thus, for such drug-resistant types take Oregacyn, 2 or 3 capsules three or more times daily. For tough conditions take the Oregacyn six times daily (with food or juice).

Survival is also dependent upon the proper diet. The diet must be high in protein. The ideal protein sources are organic milk, whole organic eggs, organic beef/lamb, and nuts/seeds. Whole unprocessed milk is the most valuable source of protein and helps greatly strengthen TB patients. A vegetable-based diet alone is insufficient, since protein is needed for tissue repair. Beta carotene-rich foods are also helpful. The top sources of this nutrient include sweet potatoes, pumpkin, squash, red sweet peppers, cantaloupe, carrots, apricots, pimentos, paprika, spinach, dandelion greens, and spirulina. There is a special natural tonic which is rich in green-source beta carotene. It is also rich in high quality vegetable protein. Known as Wild Green Powerdrops, it is highly valuable for regeneration, especially in tuberculosis. Take two dropperfuls twice daily under the tongue. For tough cases take more, like four to six dropperfuls twice daily.

There is yet another technique for aggressively treating this disease. It is the topical essential oil scrub. Using the Maximum Strength oil of wild Oreganol, rub it up and down the spine and also over the spinal muscles. Also, rub it over the big boney regions, such as the top of the thighs and shin bones. Do this at night and then cover with warm heavy blankets. This will induce sweating, which aids in the destruction of this germ.

When flying or traveling in crowded environments, such as subways, take protective cautions. If possible, wear a dust mask. Apply a few drops of oil of wild Oreganol and oil of wild lavender. Or, apply these drops on a handkerchief or Kleenex and inhale repeatedly. Also, take the oil under the tongue, a few drops as often as possible. This will largely prevent the contraction of TB in mass transit systems. Spray the Germ-a-Clenz about you wherever you go. It will help prevent disease from striking you, while protecting even the strangers near you.

Valley fever (Coccidiomycoses)

This is a desert or southwestern infection caused by the fungus Coccidiodes immitis. It only exists in certain parts of southern California, Arizona, New Mexico, and Texas. Mexico is another hotbed for this infection. It is usually not found in northern Texas. Thus, this fungus thrives only in hot dry regions, and its spores exist on dust or dry vegetation. It is carried mainly by rodents. It attacks primarily the lungs.

Millions of individuals living in the Southwest may unknowingly contract this disease. In other words there may be millions of asymptomatic carriers. When it attacks, it may commonly be confused with the flu. It develops from inhaling dust, which contains the spores. The inhalation of spores may not immediately result in active infection. It may strike later if the individual is under stress or suffers from diminished immunity. However, if a symptomatic infection occurs, it develops about one to two weeks after inhaling the dust. Respiratory symptoms are the primary feature. However, in a small percentage skin lesions and joint pain develop. If untreated, it may result in chronic diseases, including chronic fatigue syndrome, fibromyalgia, chronic lung disease, sinus syndromes, sinus headaches, and arthritis. An individual who visits the Southwest and later, for instance, within a month or two, becomes deathly ill may well have developed coccidiodes infection.

Treatment protocol

Oregacyn is a potent nutritional supplement for this condition. Take two or more capsules twice daily. Also, take P73 oil of wild oregano, five to ten drops under the tongue twice daily. For severe infections increase this to twenty drops two or three times daily. Also, to improve blood flow in the lungs take edible oil of rosemary, 10 drops twice daily. Respira Clenz is also a potent extract for the lungs. Take 10 drops twice daily. In the room of the sickened spray Germ-a-Clenz once or twice daily.

Whooping cough

This is an infection which afflicts the throat, bronchial tubes, and lungs. It is characterized by bizarre bouts of coughing, with a whoop-like sound. It is caused by a bacteria known as *Bordetella pertussis*, which is why the disease is also known as pertussis.

Pertussis is easily spread and usually occurs in children, although adults are far from immune. Americans are immunized against pertussis. However, outbreaks are occurring even in immunized individuals.

Symptoms usually begin as a cold-like syndrome, followed in a few days by a cough that is a series of short, quick coughs succeeded by a whooping-like noise, that is a long drawn out crowing sound. This "whoop" is caused by deep inspiration while the vocal cords are tightened. This is usually repeated several times, and the attack often ends with the expulsion of thick or sticky mucus. It may also end with vomiting, which occurs because of the tremendous pressure of the cough. The disease is curable and is rarely fatal. While extremely rare, serious complications may occur, like pneumonia. However, hospitalization, largely out of fear, is common.

Treatment protocol

Potent spice extracts are the ideal natural tonic for this illness. Such extracts help cleanse mucous plugs, while killing noxious invaders. Take Oregacyn, one or two capsules three times daily. During an attack open the capsule and place a quarter teaspoon of the powder under the tongue. Let this melt, and repeat every 15 minutes or so. Be sure to keep the room of the sufferer well ventilated. Also, take P73 oil of wild oregano, two or more drops under the tongue several times daily. This alone should eliminate the cough. In infants simply rub the oil on the feet or chest; it isn't necessary to give it internally. Also, for sick children also give raw honey, a tablespoon twice daily. The most potent and unprocessed types are the Mediterranean mountain honeys. These are 100% wild and raw. Of these the wild oregano honey is ideal. Wild true honeys are completely safe for use in children and even babies. For more information call 1-800-243-5242.

Chapter 5

Staying Healthy

Today, it is a challenge to stay healthy. From the point of view of overall health this is perhaps the most dangerous time in history. In general medical science is doing a poor job of helping people remain healthy and an even poorer job of helping them cure their conditions. For instance, the majority of chronic diseases, such as cancer, diabetes, high blood pressure, heart disease, lupus, arthritis, fibromyalgia, chronic fatigue syndrome, asthma, multiple sclerosis, Alzheimer's disease, Parkinson's disease, ALS, and numerous others, are increasing in incidence, not decreasing. Thus, it is crucial to determine the true cause of these illnesses as well as their natural cures.

It takes effort to maintain strong health. Yet, this is perhaps the most critical effort anyone can make. This is because the health of the body is the basis of all activity, productivity, inventiveness, and even spirituality.

The power of systematic exercise

Exercise is a powerful and effective medicine for the lungs. A lack of exercise leads to lung congestion and, thus, the accumulation of toxins.

Systematic exercise is the ideal type for lung health. This means adhering to a routine. However, it is unnecessary to perform heavy exercise. These gentle methods are equally as effective for health maintenance as harsh exercise or aerobics. A simple one or two mile walk, if done regularly, is sufficient. So is regular swimming or bicycling. Jogging is acceptable, that is if it is done on soft surfaces and if it is away from heavily polluted regions, like busy roadsides. However, walking is by far the most ideal lung-healthy exercise. This is because it is highly relaxing, and, thus, it allows time for deep breathing. It also allows for enjoyment of beautiful countryside, which is relaxing to the central nervous system. It is the central nervous system which controls breathing. It is critical for the nervous system to be healthy and relaxed in order for the lungs to be as healthy as possible. Calisthenics are also an excellent exercise. Callanetics, named after author and fitness expert, Callan Pinckney, are also highly effective. This system greatly tones the spinal and hip muscles, quickly resulting in improved lung function. Callanetics are an ideal type of exercise for strengthening the muscles needed for proper breathing. To discover more about this invaluable system check your local bookstore for the book, *Callanetics.*

Improved posture

Poor posture has particularly derogatory effects upon lung function. The lungs are closely connected to the spine. Any alteration in position or disruption in spinal anatomy negatively affects them.

Check your posture frequently. Look in the mirror. Are you hunched over? Are you constantly slouching? Is your back excessively bowed? All of these abnormal positions greatly impede lung function. If this postural dysfunction is prolonged, respiratory symptoms, as well as disease, will develop.

Improved posture often results in an immediate improvement of health. If the posture has been poor for a prolonged period, postural exercise may be required. What's more, proper chiropractic or osteopathic care often results in improved posture.

Deep breathing

Healthy posture is directly connected to the ability to breathe deeply. If the posture is poor, it is impossible to breathe normally and deeply. Every day carefully assess your posture by reviewing your standing and sitting postures in a mirror. Make a conscious effort to correct any imbalances. Keep your spine erect and draw in your abdomen. Constantly work on improving your posture. As a result you will experience a dramatic improvement in health.

Start your deep breathing program right away. You can do it on your own. Take a deep breath and exhale slowly. Repeatedly taking deep breaths will force you to stand and sit taller. It is impossible to take deep breaths if you are in a slouched position. This deep breathing will stretch the rib cage, which will ultimately help improve both your sitting and standing postures.

It is critical to make an effort to breathe correctly. Relax your abdominal muscles. Do relaxing exercises, like gentle stretching or body shaking. Loosen up. Being uptight is the greatest cause for restricted breathing. Once you relax, you can breathe fully and deeply. Breathe in to the count of four. Hold the breath for the count of four, then exhale slowly to the count of four. Do this exercise as often as possible. This deep breathing technique is described in the book *Smoke Enders* and is used successfully for aborting cigarette addiction.

Whenever possible consciously take deep breaths. The result will be a dramatic improvement in overall health.

Proper ventilation

For the purposes of human health proper ventilation means the movement of fresh air through indoor facilities. Stagnant air inside of buildings is a major cause of human disease. There is actually a science to the proper flow of air inside of buildings, which is rarely taken into account when modern buildings are built. The editors of the *Modern Home Physician*, published in 1947, describe this dilemma thusly: "If...access of air to dwellings is prevented by their being crowded together or anything prevents its passage through the dwellings, *ill health is bound to follow* (italics mine)." In other words, air must constantly circulate. Stale or stagnant air concentrates toxic fumes and microbes, which, when inhaled, results in illness.

Many people are concerned about opening windows, because they feel they are sensitive to a draught. They might believe the draught would cause them to become ill, for instance, to catch cold. There may be some truth to this concern. However, proper ventilation, in fact, prevents disease. For this the correct method is to open one or more windows widely. Opening windows partially causes draughts, which forces the air in at an abnormal rate. In other words, the rapid movement of the air is what causes the chill, not the cold air itself. Thus, if two or more windows are opened widely in the facility, draughts are prevented. In other words open the storm doors or windows completely, not just a mere slit. Don't open a door partially; open it widely. Plus, counter balance the open door or window with another one on the opposite side. This will help solve problems of air sensitivity and/or chilling.

Adrenal weakness: its role in respiratory disorders

The adrenal glands play an instrumental role in respiratory health. They are the primary defense against allergy and toxic chemical inhalation. They also help maintain normal blood flow, which is crucial for proper oxygen delivery. What's more they are needed to modulate the harsh effects of cold or winter air. If the strength of the adrenals fails, the health of the lungs will also fail. In fact, weakened adrenal glands greatly increase the risks for lung disorders.

The adrenal glands are essential for fighting allergic reactions. They produce the natural steroids needed to ward off irritations and inflammation. These steroids include natural cortisone, which is a potent anti-inflammatory agent. Thus, individuals who suffer from severe respiratory allergies are adrenally insufficient. Millions of molecules of such steroids are produced by the adrenal glands everyday. Their purpose is to ward off toxic or stressful insults, including allergic reactions.

There are a number of causes for reduced adrenal gland function. Stress greatly depletes these glands. So does poor nutrition. In fact, stress is the primary way these glands are distrusted. A high intake of sugar causes the depletion of cortisone reserves. Alcohol also destroys cortisone. The regular use of cortisone-containing drugs, including topical agents and inhalers, quickly depletes these glands.

There are hundreds of signs and symptoms of adrenal exhaustion. The wide range of symptoms is due to the diverse effects which adrenal hormones have on the body systems. Such hormones are needed for the proper function of all cells and organs. Common symptoms include fatigue, irritability, anxiety, mood swings, headaches, vague digestive complaints, an ache in the middle back, sweaty feet or palms, nervousness, insomnia, compulsive behavior, clumsiness, crying spells, muscular weakness, panic attacks, poor appetite, upper back or neck pain, heart palpitations, and alternating diarrhea and constipation. Frequently, adrenally-insufficient individuals have extreme food or beverage cravings, usually for chocolate, sugar, and/or salt. Such individuals may also have extreme cravings for alcohol, however, usually this substance makes them direly ill. Many are also addicted to coffee, which they rely on for temporary energy. If the coffee is removed, their energy plummets.

Boosting adrenal function greatly improves the body's ability to withstand the everyday stress of daily living. This benefit is also of great value with asthma, which is a stress response indicating poor adrenal reserve. By building up the adrenal capacity, the asthma gradually improves. The role of the adrenals is so critical that virtually any lung condition will benefit from improving their function: even emphysema and lung cancer. The fact is lung conditions can largely be prevented by keeping these glands vital and strong.

Certain nutritional supplements and/or herbs may help enhance adrenal function. Perhaps the most powerful of all is royal jelly. This is because royal jelly is a type of natural steroid source. In fact, this bee product contains as many as 55 different natural steroids. The steroids in royal jelly are non-toxic.

A natural and fortified royal jelly is available. Called Royal Kick, it is a stabilized and fortified royal jelly of high potency. Fortified with extra pantothenic acid and crude natural vitamin C, this is a particularly potent formula. In my experience this formula is far superior to the commercial types in terms of the clinical response seen in patients. In other words, it provides dependable results for maintaining excellent adrenal health.

How to strengthen the adrenal glands

The function of these glands can be greatly boosted. Certain vitamins are needed for adrenal steroid synthesis. The main ones are vitamin D, vitamin A, pantothenic acid, and vitamin C. To increase the strength of these glands take a natural vitamin A and D source, like cod liver oil, about a half teaspoon daily (Note: infants or children should not take this amount). Also, take a natural vitamin C source, like Flavin-C or Potent-C, about 200 mg daily. If using Potent-C take one dropperful under the tongue three times daily. Royal jelly is a superb tonic for the adrenals. This is because this substance contains up to 55 different adrenal hormones and it is easy to digest and absorb. Plus, in contrast to synthetic cortisone/steroids it is completely non-toxic. Take a crude high grade royal jelly capsule, such as Royal Kick, about 4 to 6 capsules in the a.m. daily. The latter contains some pantothenic acid, about 100 mg per capsule. For exceptionally weak adrenals increase the dose, for instance, 4 caps twice daily. Also, in certain cases megadoses of pantothenic acid may be needed. I have prescribed as much as 1000 mg of a powdered pantothenic acid capsule two or three times daily as a natural means to bolster cortisone production. This vitamin is free of significant side effects, although high doses could cause loose stools. The fact is high dose pantothenic acid is an excellent remedy for constipation. So is royal jelly. The regular intake strengthens the tone of the abdominal muscles as well as the colonic muscles.

Drug toxicity: a cause of respiratory symptoms

In order to keep the respiratory system as healthy as possible it is crucial to avoid the use of drugs. Numerous drugs may induce respiratory symptoms. In fact, many are respiratory poisons. Thus, a lung, sinus, or bronchial condition may develop strictly as a drug side effect. Cough, especially a dry type, is perhaps the most common type. High blood pressure drugs commonly cause this, particularly the so-called ACE inhibitors. Recently, it was found that the dry cough caused by these drugs is somehow related to iron deficiency. Giving iron reverses the cough. Thus, if you are taking medications and suddenly develop respiratory symptoms, see your doctor in order to reduce the dosage or, preferably, eliminate the drugs.

Keep the air healthy: the powers of Germ-a-Clenz

Germ-a-Clenz is a special solution of essential oils for cleansing the air. It is highly useful for making home or work safe by keeping the air as "microbially purified" as possible. It does so without chemicals: only pure unprocessed essential oils are used. Thus, Germ-a-Clenz dramatically enhances air quality.

The majority of commercially available essential oil-based "air purifiers" are fraudulent. They contain synthetic chemicals as well as chemically processed essential oils.

Germ-a-Clenz is exceptionally useful for cleansing the air and preventing respiratory infections. Its value is obvious during the winter and summer, when indoor air can become stagnant. Simply spray this wonderfully aromatic solution into the air once or twice daily, or spray the Germ-a-Clenz into a humidifier or vaporizer. Spray furnace/air conditioner filters frequently to decrease mold and viral transmission. Also, spray it around vents or any other region where air flows. Pump spray the air in restrooms, the hotbed for germs, on a regular basis. Today, largely due to global warming, there is a mold and fungus epidemic. Germ-a-Clenz can control or eliminate this problem. Germ-a-Clenz is available in two forms: a spray bottle and a two ounce dropper bottle.

We live in a highly toxic, polluted world. The air is foul, and so is the food. While the options are rather limited, there is no reason to give up hope. There are answers, and those answers are found in nature. If nature is relied upon and the use of synthetic chemicals is curbed, this world can be saved.

Spice extracts, such as Oreganol and Oregamax, offer tremendous hope and value for victims of lung and respiratory disorders. Modern medicine offers little or no hope, especially for individuals with chronic diseases. What's more, medical therapies have significant side effects. Furthermore, drugs fail to cure chronic respiratory conditions. In contrast, there are no serious side effects from the use of properly produced, natural spice extracts. The only issue is that in large doses it may be necessary to also take healthy bacteria, since any germicide is capable of killing healthy as well as pathogenic bacteria. Even so, spices are foods and, therefore, are completely edible. Long used as medicines, they are far safer than drugs as well as medicinal non-edible herbs such as goldenseal, ginseng, and gotu kola. Plus, in contrast to many over-the-counter respiratory medicines and weak commercial herbs, spice extracts are highly effective. Results are often noticed in minutes. If you are skeptical, you may only be hurting yourself. Thus, by denying yourself the most potent treatment known you may end up sick a lot longer than necessary. These extracts are potent germicides, and they don't discriminate: they kill, every germ known to humankind. These extracts are ideal for reversing respiratory conditions. They can also greatly bolster overall health. Take advantage of these gifts of almighty God. Your life may depend upon it.

Chapter 6

Conclusion

The respiratory system is the most vulnerable of all systems to germ or toxic invasions. It represents direct access to the internal and potentially vulnerable tissues. A mere breath can give life. However, it can also bring disease—even death.

The health of the respiratory system is dependent upon numerous factors: healthy lifestyle, proper diet, proper hygiene, and, of course, clean air. While the latter may be difficult to achieve, air can be cleansed, through the appropriate filters, aerosols, and purifiers.

Invariably, the lungs and other respiratory organs require significant biological and chemical support. This is merely to maintain optimal health. Air pollution greatly damages these tissues, lowering their resistance to disease. The lungs are highly delicate. They are readily damaged by toxic insults. The fact is such insults surround us.

Attempts must be made to keep the lungs in as clean, that is toxin-free, a condition as possible. This cannot be achieved with proper diet and exercise alone. Proper diet, nutritional supplements, herbal medicines, and detoxification programs directly improve respiratory health. Thus, only through natural, non-toxic methods can the respiratory system be healed. If no effort is made, the toxins accumulate, causing damage as well as disease. Vitamins, minerals, antioxidants, herbal extracts, spice extracts, and medicinal foods, like honey and vinegar, are powerful tools for regenerating the lungs and keeping them as healthy as possible. In other words, only natural cures are capable of reversing lung diseases. Plus, natural cures are safe, that is they will not destroy lung or respiratory tissues. Nor will they cause annoying side effects, which plague drug users.

Today, we live in an incredibly toxic world. Adding to the toxicity by taking harsh drugs will diminish health. The effort should be made to reduce the intake of harsh medications, relying on the more gentle yet powerful natural medicines, which will not cause organ toxicity. Consider the use of honey and vinegar or oil of wild oregano. These natural medicines are effective yet utterly non-toxic. Plus, in contrast to pharmaceutical drugs they fail to pollute the environment.

This is why nutritional and herbal supplements are the answer for enhancing respiratory health. They strengthen the lungs. They help cleanse the sinuses. They purge poisons from the tonsils. They keep the lung and sinus passages open. They prevent germs from attacking the respiratory passages. Plus, they aid the body in the removal of toxins and in the destruction of germs. What's more, many of these natural cures are germicidal, meaning they destroy germs. The fact is natural germicides, such as oil of wild oregano, destroy microbes virtually on contact. This is why such agents are of lifesaving importance for respiratory conditions. The fact is the daily intake of natural antiseptics can help overall health dramatically by curtailing the incidence of respiratory infections. Many of these natural substances are powerful enough to prevent any type of respiratory infection, including the diabolical ones likely to cause the soon -to-strike pandemics.

Prevention is the key for maintaining a strong, healthy body. Respiratory infections are dangerous, and there may be no guarantee that the infection can be cured, especially if treatment begins too late. However, in general the natural antiseptics are so powerful, so valuable, that they will help virtually at any stage in the infection. This is because these antiseptics are capable of killing in minutes: in fact, seconds. At least they will help prevent fatality. At a minimum they will ease agony and pain. Thus, a thorough knowledge of what is needed for such protection is crucial in order to prevent serious illness.

Spice extracts offer germicidal power unknown in the drug kingdom. Furthermore, spices are well respected for their diversity of effects upon the respiratory system. They help keep the respiratory passages open, decreasing mucus or thinning it. They neutralize the toxicity of allergens. They boost the ability of the immune system to eliminate germs. Plus, they destroy noxious germs. They have been proven effective by the latest scientific studies. What's more, they have been proven to kill a wide range of germs, including medically impossible types such as drug-resistant staph and TB. Spice oils, such as the combination found in Oregacyn, have proven highly effective, even against anthrax. Tests at the EPA have proven that the oils found in Oregacyn are the only natural compounds capable of destroying this germ. Thus, these oils are effective for reversing virtually all respiratory illnesses.

Plagues will happen. Chronic diseases, which plague humanity, already exist. This book predicts the onset of major plagues, which could devastate all of humankind. For instance, according to *Mother Jones* unless the appropriate defenses are created it is inevitable that tuberculosis will sweep this country. The predictions are that each year it could kill tens of thousands of Americans. Thus, it is necessary to prepare for the worst. If used systematically, the information in this book could save thousands, perhaps millions, of lives. Plus, it could give vibrant life to the already living.

Appendix

Foods or Food Additives that May Act as Respiratory Poisons

- food dyes, especially Yellow Dye # 5 (tartrazine)
- refined sugar
- nitrated/processed meats
- wheat or wheat germ
- cow's milk, including non-fat and skim
- peanuts and peanut butter
- baker's and brewer's yeast
- chocolate
- eggs and/or egg protein (includes infant formulas)
- soy and soy milk
- malt and barley
- seafood (especially lobster, shrimp, crab, and oysters)
- bottom-dwelling fish, including flounder and sole
- aspartame (NutraSweet)

Foods or Food Additives Likely to Cause Sinus Problems

- aspartame
- Yellow Dye # 5 (tartrazine)
- butter
- wheat and wheat germ
- peanuts and peanut butter

- eggs

- cheese

- chocolate

- cream or cream cheese

- cow's milk

- fruit drinks

- soda pop

- refined sugar

- citrus juice (in some instances, especially the highly processed types)

- soy and soy milk

Foods which Enhance Respiratory Functions

- rosemary

- oregano

- ginger

- caraway

- cumin

- mustard

- basil

- sage

- thyme

- pumpkin seeds and pumpkinseed oil (as a source of natural fatty acids), zinc (in the seeds), and phospholipids

- fresh citrus juice (as a rich source of vitamin C)

- spinach

- radishes

- wasabi and/or horseradish

- broccoli

- egg yolks (as a source of phospholipids)

- garlic

- onion

- beef broth

- chicken broth

- nuts and seeds

- fresh red meat (as a source of amino acids and phospholipids)

- organic liver (as a source of vitamin A and phospholipids)

- pumpkin and squash (as a source of vitamin A in the form of beta carotene)

- sweet potatoes (as a source of vitamin A in the form of beta carotene)

- halibut and salmon (as a source of fatty fish oils and phospholipids, as well as animal-source vitamin A)

- herring and sardines (as a source of fatty fish oils and vitamin A)

- cheddar and Swiss cheese

- hot chili peppers

- parsley (as a source of magnesium)

- beet and turnip greens (as a source of vitamin A in the form of beta carotene)

- nettles

- dandelion
- rose hips

Foods or Food Additives Likely to Provoke Asthma Attacks

- yellow dye # 5 (tartrazine)

- baker's and brewer's yeast

- cow's milk and/or cow's milk cheese

- wheat

- malt or barley

- corn or corn starch

- red or white wine

- colored alcoholic beverages

- refined vegetable oils (any type)

- brominated vegetable oils

- hydrogenated vegetable oils

- partially hydrogenated vegetable oils

- lard

- cottonseed meal or oil

- MSG

Bibliography

Anderson, W. A. D. 1960. *Synopsis of Pathology*. St. Louis: C. V. Mosby Co.

Birkeland, Jorgen. 1949. *Microbiology and Man*. New York: Appleton-Century-Crofts.

Evans, W. A. 1917. *How to Keep Well*. New York: D. Appelton and Co.

The Editors. *Our Human Body*. Pleasantville, NY: Reader's Digest.

Fishbein, M. 1956. *Modern Home Medical Adviser*. New York: Garden City Books.

Haas, F. and S. Haas.1990. *The Chronic Bronchitis and Emphysema Handbook*. New York: John Wiley & Sons.

Harris, A. and M. Super. 1995. *Cystic Fibrosis: the Facts*. Oxford: Oxford Univ. Press.

Introduction to Respiratory Diseases. 1969. National Tuberculosis and Respiratory Disease Association.

Lindlar, V. H. 1943. *Most Popular Foreign Dishes*. New York: Journal of Living Publ.

Lorand, A. 1928. *Health Through Rational Diet*. Philadelphia: F. A. Davis Co.

Fishbein, M. 1970. *Medical and Health Encyclopedia: V. 18*. New York: H. S. Stuttman Co.

Robinson, V. 1947. *The New Modern Home Physician*. New York: Wm. Wise & Co.

Seltzer, A. 1949. *Your Nasal Sinuses and Their Disorders*. New York: Froben Press.

Smith, W.H. 1884. *The Human Body and Its Health*. New York: American Book Co.

Weinstein, A. 1987. *Asthma*. St. Louis: McGraw-Hill.

Index

Exocrine glands, 93-94

F

Family Health Guide, 51
Family Physician and Home Book of Health, 159
Fatigue, 65, 71, 87, 109, 169, 173, 177, 182
Fatty acids, 29, 70, 90, 95, 116, 141, 192
Fish, 70, 90, 96, 141-142, 191, 193
Fishbein, Dr. Morris, 61
Fistulas, 141, 169
Flavin-C, 60, 67, 70, 74, 90, 101, 105, 114, 119-120, 138, 161, 170, 183
Flavonoids, 87, 91, 103, 120, 161 *see also* Bioflavonoids
Flu, 1, 5, 8, 10, 35, 40, 47-48, 55, 80, 84, 86-87, 105-112, 115, 123-124, 129, 173
Food allergies, 31, 38-41
Food allergy tests, 42 *see also* Food intolerance test
Food Intolerance Test, 42-43
Forgetfulness, 38
Foster, Irving, 80
Foxglove, 159
Fudenberg, Dr. H., 109

Full spectrum lights, 170
Fungal infections, 36, 66, 71, 73, 107, 115-116, 135, 137, 148, 166 *see also* Candida albicans

G

Garlic, 44, 55, 101, 161, 193
Gases, 7, 16-18, 25-26, 82, 86
Germ-A-Clenz, 50, 77, 127-128, 131, 134, 150, 154, 161, 173-174, 185
Global warming, 7, 185
Gluten-containing grains, 97
Grapefruit, 67, 77, 101, 134
Greer, Dr. J. H., 51, 53, 154-155
Guava, 119

H

Hanson, L. E., 160
Hantavirus, 10
Hay fever, 5, 38, 112-114
Headaches, 27, 36-37, 41, 43, 53, 86, 123, 147, 149, 152, 173, 182
Health Through Rational Diet, 88
Health-Bac, 51, 62
Healthy bacteria, 36, 51, 62, 112, 186
Hemoglobin, 15
Hemophilus influenzae, 110-111
Hemorrhage, 152

Books and Cassettes

#1   *How to Eat Right and Live Longer*—$21.95
373 pages   6 x 9 inch softbound   ISBN 0911119213

Dr. Ingram's most comprehensive book on diet and nutrition. Describes the treatment of a wide range of illnesses through diet and nutritional supplementation. Emphasis is on the nutritional treatment of heart disease, high cholesterol, high triglycerides, diabetes, obesity, allergies, arthritis, neurological disorders, and alcoholism. Step-by-step nutritional protocols, dietary instruction, personalized nutritional/blood analysis, and 100 recipes included.

#2   *Self-Test Nutrition Guide*—$24.95
330 pages   5 1/2 x 8 1/2 inch softbound   ISBN 0911119053

Test yourself to determine your nutritional deficiencies from *A to zinc*. Other tests show evidence of possible health problems such as adrenal insufficiency, chemical toxicity, thyroid insufficiency, intestinal malabsorption, liver dysfunction, and premature aging. Sugar, caffeine, sulfite, food dye, and MSG overload also evaluated. Each test followed by specific and thorough nutritional recommendations. Find out what you are lacking.

#3   *Who Needs Headaches?*—$13.95
158 pages   6 x 9 inch softbound   ISBN 0911119329

A nutritional approach to solving the migraine dilemma. Emphasizes food allergies, nutritional deficiencies, and hormonal disturbances and how to diagnose them as well as how to reverse them nutritionally. Chapter on structural therapy for tension headaches included.

#4   *Tea Tree Oil: the Natural Antiseptic*—$12.95
119 pages   5 1/2 x 8 1/2 inch softbound   ISBN 0911119493

Some things need to be killed: bacteria, viruses, fungi, parasites, and parasitic insects. Learn how to battle infectious disease with tea tree oil, one of Nature's most versatile and potent antiseptics. Information particularly valuable for homemakers, travelers, wilderness buffs, fishermen, and athletes.

#5   *How to Survive Disasters with Natural Medicines*—$13.95
137 pages   5 1/2 x 8 1/2 inch softbound   ISBN 0911119442

Natural disasters, toxic waste spills, fires, parasite infestations, accidents, radiation leakage, and water contamination all demand immediate action. Learn to deal with both major and minor disasters using only natural remedies which are both safe and effective. Destroy ticks, stop wound infection, end the pain of toothache, neutralize animal/insect bites, abort diarrhea and/or dysentery, treat burns/cuts — all with natural substances.

#6   *Supermarket Remedies for Better Health*—$29.95
325 pages   6 1/4 x 9 1/4 inch hardbound   ISBN 0911119647

Reverse health problems with foods, herbs, and spices. Learn to shop for your ailments at the supermarket, health store, and farmer's market. A supermarket juice that reverses heart disease, a vegetable that halts depression, a berry which eliminates stomach aches, a fruit which lowers cholesterol, a berry for poor vision, a protein for great energy, a spice which kills germs and much more. Use supermarket remedies for hundreds of ailments.

#7 *The Cure is in the Cupboard: How to Use Oregano for Better Health*—$19.95
203 pages–Revised Edition 5 1/2 x 8 1/2 inch softback ISBN 0911119744
Oregano helps you regain your health and then stay healthy. This is what saved Dr. Ingram's life. Learn how to use oregano and its essential oil for fighting infection and eliminating pain. Combat skin disorders, injuries, wounds, and dental problems. Particularly valuable for fungal infections.

#8 *Lifesaving Cures*—$19.95
312 pages, 6x 9 inch softback ISBN 1931078009
To survive in the 21st century you must know lifesaving cures. This book describes the most powerful remedies for reversing everyday illnesses. With this book of natural cures Dr. Ingram provides hundreds of natural answers for dozens of ailments.

#9 *The Respiratory Solution*—$14.95
206 pages, 5.5x 8.5 inch softback ISBN 1931078076
Learn the most powerful natural cures for reversing dozens of respiratory ailments. Gain fast relief from sinus problems, allergies, mold, bronchial problems, colds, flu and much more using edible natural foods and herbs.

#10 *The Longevity Solution*—$12.95
144 pages, 5.5x 8.5 inch softback ISBN 1931078017
A book that explains the incredible powers of royal jelly. Reverse fatigue, hormonal problems, hot flashes, anxiety, depression, insomnia, irritability, panic attacks, and much more. Stall the aging process with royal jelly.

Cassette Tapes and Programs

#1 *How to Use Oregano for Common Illnesses*—$10.00
A must for oregano lovers. Contains detailed information not found in the book. Specific protocols for dozens of illnesses and diseases plus case histories. Learn hundreds of uses for wild oregano oil and herb—from the Doctor himself.

#2 *Professional/Advanced Series*—$85.00* *The Warning Signs of Nutritional Deficiency 4 tapes Manual: 100 pages, with Judy Kay Gray, M. S.*
Master Dr. Ingram's knowledge about nutritional deficiency and natural medicine. Find out how to discern your specific deficiencies; become proficient in spotting nutritional deficiencies in others. Includes lifesaving information on the treatment of disease with nutritional medicine. Become an expert.

#3 *Wild Oregano, Lifesaving Spice*—$9.95
Dr. Ingram's famous lecture on the power of wild oregano. Learn all the most compelling facts—why it worked, the research, and true life stories—informative and entertaining.

For ordering information call (800) 243-5242 or for overseas orders call
(847) 473-4700. To send a fax: (847) 473-4780. E-mail: droregano@aol.com
For more information about the products mentioned in this book see the Web site,
www.Oreganol.com.